I0421924

Introduction

I'm no doctor, nor do I have any kind of degree related to the subject matter of this book. As such you are welcome to judge me accordingly but, a whole lot of people have changed the world and the way you live and they did not have degrees either. So I recommend you read this booklet first, before you judge me and I think you will see that a person does not need a degree to be smart, hard working, well informed, and indeed an expert in their field.

Although the horrendously overpriced rip-off colleges have not put me hundreds of thousands of dollars in debt, I am a consumer and I found myself looking down the massive vitamins and supplements aisle of a typical drug store and realized that there was absolutely no way a person could walk up, pick a multivitamin off the shelf, and get it right.

Furthermore, I realized that there was no way anyone could pick ANY product off of those shelves and get it right – that is, try to take something that would shore up what they perceive to be their weakness. And how could a person, like myself, even know what their weaknesses were in the first place?

This series of books intends to address this problem. I have done all of the research and I can tell you exactly which products have the best ingredients – which ones work – and where appropriate, which ones have such useless ingredients in them that they are worth avoiding.

And that's an important point, it is amazing to consider that some supplements on the very shelf I mentioned are almost completely useless, and it is amazing that they are even allowed to sell the garbage at all, but they are allowed to do it and we all know exactly why: greed and the insatiable thirst to steal that almighty dollar by the millions – the same greed, in the food industry that has made us all sick in the first place!

If we all stop buying the poisons that the greedy monsters want to shove down our throats, then they will stop wasting their time manufacturing those cancer cocktails and maybe they might actually start making products that are good for us.

One in three Americans will die of cancer, a disease that was one of the rarest known to medical science prior to World War II with only a handful – and I mean LESS THAN TEN – cases diagnosed by doctors each year. In the fifties these numbers exploded exponentially from hundreds per year to thousands to tens of thousands to hundreds of thousands of new cases each year. What changed? Two things: chemical additives to the foods we eat started appearing in the fifties and the nuclear bombs were set off in the mid-forties through the seventies. These bombs create what we all know very well as the mushroom cloud, this thing sends radioactive fallout as high as 30 miles, that's the edge of space, and the upper atmospheric winds can distribute that fallout world wide and it only takes ONE RADIOACTIVE ATOM to be absorbed by you, to ultimately possibly cause cancer in you.

We have no way of protecting ourselves from the radioactive fallout of those bombs or the Chernobyl and Fukushima disasters that have easily poured ten times the radioactive contamination into the Earth's atmosphere as all of the bombs before them did, but we can stop eating the POISONS that cause cancer and we can start eating the things that will make us healthier.

Three things are killing people:

1. They eat POISON in the form of CANCER CAUSING ADDITIVES to their PROCESSED foods on a DAILY BASIS. (And they are exposed to other POISONS also on a daily basis, like DIESEL ENGINE FUMES, HARSH CLEANER FUMES, etc.)

2. POOR DIET: even if you eat good foods, an unmanaged diet consisting of nothing but natural whole foods will most likely fail to deliver everything the body needs because some nutrients are rare in the plant kingdom and only a few foods actually provide them in significant quantities. Without knowing precisely what the body needs and what foods can fulfill those needs, a person will suffer chronic deficiencies in critical nutrients which can have severe consequences to their health.

3. LACK OF EXERCISE: You cannot expect to be healthy if you do not engage in EXERCISE. Exercise is necessary for cardiovascular health and sweating is one of the methods the body uses for detoxification, therefore it is vital for OPTIMUM THRIVE-LEVEL health.

This series is designed to explain the needs of the human body and how to cover those needs in order to achieve OPTIMUM THRIVE-LEVEL health and avoid the BIG SEVEN modern deadly epidemic plagues that are killing over a MILLION people each year: 1) High Blood Pressure, 2) High Cholesterol, 3) Type II Diabetes, 4) Alzheimer's Disease, 5) Cardiovascular Disease, 6) Stroke and 7) Cancer. Why isn't "heart attack" in the Big Seven? Heart failure is most certainly in there: it is final event of High Blood Pressure, High Cholesterol and Cardiovascular Disease. It is important to know that the primary cause of ALL of these modern plagues is POOR DIET and that MOST of those deaths are PREVENTABLE.

Furthermore and of far greater importance, the series will show you how to eat properly, or rather, how to set up a regular food regimen that will provide you with all of the essential nutrients from natural whole foods rather than pills which have been shown in many studies to be far less effective than the whole foods they were extracted from or worse: pure synthetic replacements. More and more health professionals are starting to recommend natural whole foods over purified extracts and manufactured chemicals, a realization that I have been advocating for thirty years.

When it comes to cancer, anyone suffering from it certainly knows plenty more about it than I do, so the main goals of this book:

1. I am not going to attempt to describe even the major categories of cancer, much less the countless varieties called "cell lines." That information is readily available online and from your doctor. You don't really want to hear about dozens of kinds and hundreds of varieties that you DON'T HAVE anyway.

2. I will include the holistic plants that have been used traditionally for the treatment of cancer as well as those that have at least one study indicating its potential for helping to combat cancer.

3. Most plants (really the phytonutrients they contain) will target specific types of cancer, while others are more general in their effects. I will try to include as much of this relevant information as is currently available.

And TWO IMPORTANT RULES:

1. Holistic herbal medicines CANNOT POSSIBLY REPLACE or SUBSTITUTE FOR modern conventional medicine: if you even suspect you have cancer then YOU MUST SEE A DOCTOR AND FOLLOW THEIR ADVICE AND TREATMENT.

2. If you do choose to pursue "alternative medicinal treatment" NOTIFY YOUR DOCTOR of exactly what you are taking and the specific dosages you are taking.

Herbal remedies ARE NO CURE FOR CANCER AND THERE MAY NEVER BE ANY SINGLE CURE FOR CANCER which is a large CATEGORY of diseases and not a single disease. Because of this situation, some herbals have had remarkable success in HELPING CONVENTIONAL MEDICINE to defeat SPECIFIC CELL LINES of cancer while they have NO EFFECT on others. ALWAYS WORK WITH YOUR DOCTOR in the treatment of your cancer.

I don't practice holism or herbal medicine for two reasons: 1) When I give anyone a piece of advice, it is always basically a "trial and error" process, but many people are tempted to overindulge. If a little of something is good for them then they automatically figure that a lot of it must be extremely good for them and it never is. 2) It is an enormous responsibility to tell someone "Plant X will cure Ailment Y." Even if the plant has scientific studies showing this to be true, that does not mean that it will work for every individual on Earth. And giving someone that piece of information doesn't mean they will use the plant responsibly and correctly, and in many cases I would be relying on their ability to "self-diagnose" and they are not always correct as well as the fact that for serious issues they should visit their doctor first – not an herbalist.

Consequently, I generally avoid even casually mentioning the medicinal power of herbs to anybody. I do practice herbalism on myself and have so since my mother raised me on it, but if something goes wrong then I only hurt myself and have no one else to blame. However, by writing this book I am giving a lot of advice on medicinal herbs to a lot of folks and the potential for disaster is definitely higher than giving advice to friends because they know me and we can sit down and have a long discussion about their specific issue and I can cover safety in enough detail that they know the situation starting with the fact that I cannot take responsibility for the consequences of their decision to take my advice and I will not take responsibility if they misuse the remedy or if it does not work for them. Therefore, it is paramount that you understand the situation completely as well.

SAFETY WITH HERBALISM

Even the safest and most important substances needed by the human body like Oxygen and Water, can cause trouble in excess; hyperventilating will make you dizzy and drinking too much water can mess with your internal fluid osmotic pressures and cause much more trouble than you might think. So even if these top two requirements of the body can cause trouble in excess then it stands to reason that EVERYTHING will cause trouble in excess. Even the most innocuous and healthy foods can cause serious issues through overindulgence and some Vitamins and ALL of the Minerals can become toxic in excess. As a result of this it is imperative that you understand the basic rules of safety regarding proper natural source nutrition and herbalism which are one and the same.

1) DO NOT "SELF-DIAGNOSE" – Quite often people can do this and get it right, but they are just as likely to get it WRONG. And that could have DEADLY consequences: something as simple as dizziness or ringing in the ears can be signs of a life-threatening health issue. Whenever you get some new symptom out-of-the-

blue, you cannot afford to ignore it and you cannot afford to ASSUME you know what is causing it. Even doctors go to other doctors to make absolutely certain they know what's wrong before they take up a course of action to correct the issue. If they feel that this is necessary and prudent – and they studied medicine for ten years – then all of us who have not studied medicine must seek a professional diagnosis as well. IF YOU HAVE ANY UNUSUAL SYMPTOM(S) GO TO A DOCTOR FOR A PROPER DIAGNOSIS.
2) DO NOT "SELF-MEDICATE" – Under normal circumstances, such as being overweight with no overt symptoms that could be warning signs of some serious health issue, you can certainly engage in the modification of your diet - convert to what doctor's call a "proper diet" and begin to exercise in order to pursue what I call "Optimum thrive-level" health. However, when it comes to serious issues such as high blood pressure, Type II diabetes, high cholesterol, etc, then the situation is different. By the time you experience symptoms of any of these issues, they may already be advanced to the point of being life-threatening. So following rule #1 – going to a doctor – comes Rule #2 – FOLLOW THE DOCTOR'S ADVICE. As long as your issue has not progressed to the point of being dangerous, you can certainly ask your doctor if it is possible to correct the situation with proper diet and exercise rather than take harsh prescription drugs. Most conscientious doctor's would sing and dance if a patient made this suggestion and was serious about making this commitment. But there are doctor's who might insist on setting you up for a lifetime addiction to prescription drugs because they are under a lot of pressure by the drug companies to sell them and they have a huge overhead; doctors are paying hundreds of thousands of dollars a year in malpractice insurance premiums and getting you hooked on harsh drugs gets you coming back for regular checkups and prescription refills, lab tests, etc. Most simple issues like high blood pressure and high cholesterol in particular do not necessarily need to be treated with drugs and all of this additional expense. The primary cause of two maladies is poor diet and they can be fixed by proper diet.
3) DO NOT OVERINDULGE – Everyone (including myself) is tempted to over-medicate. If one pill works alright, then two must work twice as well and ten must be an instant cure, right? WRONG. Always remember: MORE IS NEVER BETTER WHEN IT COMES TO STRONG MEDICINE. As a matter of fact, more is never better when it comes to ANYTHING your body requires no matter how simple and harmless it might seem. Even some medicinal herbs offered as supplements in pill form may not be necessary in the amount indicated on the bottle. In some cases this might indeed be the correct dosage for most people, but I am not most people – no one is. And we cannot ignore the fact that the manufacturer makes money by selling the item. So the faster you run out of it, the faster you will need to buy more of it.

4) BE CAREFUL OF ALLERGIC REACTIONS – I am surprised that no herbalist ever mentions this issue and it is IMPORTANT. In fact this is another reason I don't practice herbalism and it is the main reason I don't like herbal tea blends or custom formula mixes in dietary supplements. Whenever you decide to take a natural plant-based substance for the first time, the potential for an adverse allergic reaction is very real and possibly very dangerous – ANYONE COULD HAVE A DEADLY ALLERGIC REACTION TO ANY NEW FOREIGN SUBSTANCE INTRODUCED INTO THEIR BODY AT ANY AGE. Even if you have never had an allergic reaction to anything in your life, you could still have a reaction to any new foreign substance, even a synthetic medication and each natural whole plant contains HUNDREDS of chemical constituents and you could be allergic to any one of them. If you are going to try an herbal tea for the first time; MAKE A SMALL AMOUNT OF THE SUBSTANCE TO BE TESTED AND SCRATCH YOUR SKIN WITH A NEEDLE AND PUT A DROP ON THE SCRATCH. You do not have to draw blood with the scratch – that's too deep, and you don't need a scratch any longer than the droplet either. If it swells and turns red, then you know you are allergic to this plant and you need to try something else. You do not need to do this Schick Test for topical treatments like essential oils for external use only. For those, just place a drop on the tender spot of your inner wrist (below the palm of your hand) and watch for the same reaction (swelling, redness, itching, etc.) Supplement pills can also be tested in the same way. For gelcaps just squeeze the contents onto the scratch, for dry pills crush them in a mortar and pestle, add a few drops of water, mash this up thoroughly then apply to the scratch. Even those plants that do not cause an adverse reaction to the Schick Test could still cause a bad systemic reaction after being consumed. Always try a small amount of herbal tea (no more than a tablespoon) or a single supplement gelcap or half a dry pill. Have a contingency plan if you do end up having a severe reaction. (Have someone available to give you a ride to the hospital and take the product packaging with you so the doctor knows the cause and can determine the best treatment.) NEVER TRY MORE THAN ONE NEW SUBSTANCE AT A TIME AND TRY THEM IN SMALL AMOUNTS. Give any new substance, be it an edible plant, herbal tea, or dietary supplement at least two days before adding anything else so you are sure that it is safe.
5) ALWAYS GET A SECOND OPINION – I always verify the alleged benefits of any plant, edible or medicinal, from at least two independent sources. I list my own sources in the last chapter, but this advice pertains not only to a plant's nutritional or medicinal benefits but also its safety and you should get more than one opinion concerning your own nutritional or medicinal needs. If your doctor seems too eager to get you hooked on prescription drugs – especially for high blood pressure or high cholesterol, both of

which can be controlled with proper diet and exercise – then ask another doctor. While I make every effort to verify the information I provide, typographical errors, omissions of critical details, and outright erroneous details are bound to happen not only in my sources, but in my own books as well, especially since I am not submitting these works to an editor. You have been warned: ALWAYS VERIFY ANY INFORMATION FROM ANY SOURCE ABOUT ANY SUBSTANCE YOU PLAN TO PUT INTO YOUR BODY AND ALWAYS SEEK SECOND OPINIONS CONCERNING YOUR OWN SPECIFIC AND POSSIBLY UNIQUE SITUATION.

6) NEVER MIX DRUGS – Most people forget that all plants contain hundreds of identified compounds each and some of those compounds are very potent. IF YOU ARE CURRENTLY ON ANY PRESCRIPTION DRUG YOU MUST NOT TAKE ANY HOLISTIC HERB UNTIL YOU CHECK WITH YOUR DOCTOR. Some of the harsh drugs prescribed for depression and many other drugs may be MAOI's (Monoamine Oxidase Inhibitors.) The problem is that Grapefruit also contains MAOI's which is why people on certain medications are warned to avoid this simple common fruit. As such if you are currently on ANY medication you MUST check with your doctor before adding any new plant to your dietary or supplement intake. The vast majority of holistic plants, edible or medicinal, do not have adverse reactions in combinations because they are not concentrated like prescription drugs but, there are exceptions to this generally accepted rule like Coleus. The active compound, Forskolin, is very potent medicine (it is a strong immune stimulant) and people in generally good health should take it very sparingly regardless of any other natural whole foods or holistic herbs they might be taking. However, I do believe in the "Shotgun effect." That is, rather than depend on one remedy to treat a given issue, use many different remedies but not all at once. In other words, if you want to improve your immune system, take Coleus one day, Cat's Claw the next day, Astragalus the next, Eleuthero the next, and so on. By taking a different plant each day, you are ensuring that you get many different powerful phytonutrients, all of which promote increased immune system function in different ways which add up to make the immune system even stronger than any one holistic herb could. And at the same time you are avoiding overindulgence in any one of them and also helping to avoid MIXING them all at once which could have an adverse reaction. It's not ideal though because many phytonutrients are steroids which simply means that they act like hormones: they trigger our cells to begin behaving in a different way. Rather than actively participate directly toward some desired effect, they tell our own cells to start producing the desired effect. So these can have long-lasting and potent effects and these can have adverse reactions over the long-term. This is why I never recommend remedial plants to be taken daily or over long periods of time. The ultimate goal is to be healthy which starts with proper diet and getting all of the "Big 43 Essential Nutrients" (discussed in detail in "Getting the Big 43 Essential Nutrients The Natural Way, Vol.") Beyond that, you must endeavor to always consume the greatest variety of foods and medicinal herbs as possible from one day to the next. This ensures that you will be exposed to the greatest selection of phytochemicals found in those foods, many of which may eventually turn out to be just as essential as those that have already been identified (the "Big 43" essential nutrients.) Since the goal is OPTIMUM THRIVE-LEVEL health and wellness, IF YOU FEEL "OUT OF SORTS" OR A NOTICEABLE SYMPTOM, when you never had such an issue before trying these foods and holistic herbs, then the best response is to, STOP ALL MEDICINAL HERBS IMMEDIATELY AND SEE YOUR DOCTOR.

7) WORK WITH YOUR DOCTOR – It may be necessary to find an open-minded doctor who is much more knowledgeable about the holistic herbs. Many doctors are beginning to embrace these plants because they are a subcategory of the Natural Whole Food Diet which they have all been recommending since the 1970's when people began eating more processed and packaged foods laced with CANCER CAUSING CHEMICALS than natural whole foods. But there are still many doctors who are unfamiliar with medicinal plants and very skeptical of their efficacy and safety and they will obviously always oppose anything you might wish to try. Far be it from me to suggest that the doctors are wrong, all I am saying is that no doctor would ever suggest that your diet should consist solely of Twinkies (completely synthetic food) and they simply have far too much faith in manufactured medicines. Also no doctor can cannot deny that the vast majority of all prescription drugs were discovered in plants first (salicylic acid or "Aspirin" was discovered in Willow Bark Tea used by Native Americans for aches and pains.) If you have been diagnosed with any serious condition such as kidney disease, liver disease, cancer, etc, you must FOLLOW YOUR DOCTOR'S ADVICE AND TREATMENT. The "Natural Whole Foods and Holistic Herbs Diet" is intended to take you away from a poor diet and toward a superior healthy and nutritious one and TO AUGMENT YOUR DOCTOR'S ADVICE AND TREATMENT BUT NEVER TO REPLACE OR SUPERCEDE THOSE EFFORTS.

IF YOU SUSPECT THAT YOU HAVE CANCER: SEE YOUR DOCTOR AND FOLLOW THEIR ADIVCE AND TREATMENT.

THERE IS NO "MIRACLE" CURE FOR CANCER. WHILE MANY PLANTS IN THIS BOOK SHOW GREAT PROMISE THEY ARE NOT SUBSTITUTES FOR CONVENTIONAL MEDICAL SCIENCE AND MODERN TREAMENTS.

When I started the research for this book I was concerned that I might not find enough material for this section. That is, I thought there would only be a few natural whole food plants and medicinal herbs that have been shown in at least one scientific study to have some positive effect on actually fighting cancer. I was wrong. In fact, I have had to abbreviate the entries for this section because it seems like there are MORE plants with anticancer properties than not. If ever there was a giant flashing neon sign on the side of a blimp telling you what you should be eating (natural whole plant foods) this list should convince you to change your diet.

I have included all plants that have shown at least some form of "anticancer" property in at least one laboratory experiment or clinical trial that are also RELATIVELY safe to consume.

To be clear, I am NOT implying that any plant from the following list will cure cancer mainly because the work has not been done to test and ultimately prove that. But, the preliminary work has been done that indicates that some of these plants MIGHT hold phytochemicals in them that COULD ultimately be developed into effective treatments and even cures. Since plenty of them are actually already on the menu (i.e. they are edible) then it doesn't hurt to include them in your daily or weekly dietary line up. And doing so could lead to improved health in general, since many of them have far more than just anticancer powers.

The *IM notation indicates that the plant is also in the Immunostimulant Plants List that follows. As always:

ALERT YOUR DOCTOR TO ANY SIGNIFICANT DIETARY CHANGES YOU MAKE, AND FOLLOW THEIR ADVICE.

1. ACEROLA (Malpighia emarginata)

Top Recommended Edible Fruit: Just ONE little berry has over 100% RDA of Vitamin C. But their power doesn't stop there; they are loaded with anthocyanidins, powerful antioxidants, that have enormous health benefits and studies have shown that Acerola targets HSC-2 and HSG cell lines, killing the cancer cells while nourishing healthy cells. Studies have also shown that the berries and juice have marked anti-inflammatory effects and demonstrate strong protective power for the liver from alcohol abuse.[20]

2. AERVA (Aerva lanata)

Recommended Holistic Herb: This is one of many small weeds that have big potential. It has been shown to be nephroprotective and helps prevent and break up kidney stones. One study showed that it has anticancer power against DAL, EAC and B16F10 cell lines. Another study showed efficacy against forms of leukemia, lung and colon cancer. [6]

3. AFRICAN SAUSAGE TREE (Kigelia africana)

Recommended Holistic Herb: Cucumber Tree is a well known

medicine in Africa and it has some potent phytochemicals in it. One study of the crude extracts of the stem bark and fruit showed cytotoxic activity against melanoma and other cancer cell lines. The major components are Norviburtinal, beta-Sitosterol, and Lapachol which has been found to be an effective treatment of skin cancer and kaposis sarcoma. Another study of the fruit showed growth inhibitory activity against human melanoma cells. Compounds isolated included Demethylkigelin, Kigelin, Oleic Acid, Hexeicosanoic Acid, 2-(1-hydroxyethyl)-naphtho[2,3-b]furan-4,9-dione (which showed cytotoxic effect against two breast cancer cell lines,) and Ferulic Acid. [21]

4. AGARICUS BLAZEI MUSHROOM *IM

Top Recommended Edible Mushroom: One of the species of mushrooms found to have amazing holistic medicinal properties, this mushroom is quite edible – considered a delicacy which means it's expensive – and now that it has been found to be loaded with beta-Glucans – a class of polysaccharides unique to mushrooms which have been shown to fight cancer – it is now outrageously expensive, but it might be very well worth it. Try to stick to the natural mushroom rather than extracts as there is some concern that those might cause liver damage.[22][74][332]

5. AGAVE (Agave americana)

Top Recommended Edible Plant By-Product: Raw Agave is toxic, but the processed syrup is not only a very good sweetener and honey substitute, it is also loaded with antioxidants and other powerful phytonutrients. One study found a new saponin along with three known saponins and Hecogenin tetraglycoside which showed cytotoxic activity against HL-60. Another study revealed that extracts display potent cytotoxicity against MCF-7 cells.[23]

6. AGRIMONY (Agrimonia eupatoria)

Top Recommended Holistic Herb: This cousin of the Rose is well known and respected in holistic natural medicine circles and has been used for centuries as a blood and liver depurative. The plant contains many compounds that have been found to have anticancer properties including: Catechin, Palmitic Acid, Quercitin, and Ursolic Acid. [27]

7. ALFALFA (Medicago sativa) *IM

Top Recommended Edible Plant: Limit your exposure to Alfalfa; either whole leaves and young shoots or alfalfa sprouts in a salad once a week. Alfalfa contains lectins that have been shown to be detrimental to human health. However, its health benefits cannot be ignored either and it is believed to have anticancer properties amongst other health benefits including lowering blood sugar and cholesterol levels and acting as a strong immunostimulant.[19]

8. ALLAMANDA (Allamanda cathartica)

TOXIC: This hardy and popular perennial ornamental bush is well known for its large yellow lily-like flowers. The leaf decoctions were popularized long ago as a strong purgative and the plant has since been verified to have several health promoting properties including anticancer power. One study showed an antiproliferative effect against the K562 cell line.[29]

9. ALOE (Aloe vera) *IM

Top Recommended Holistic Herb: Aloe vera's healing power is legendary, but in chronic excess (taken internally) it can become toxic. Pills are fine but there was one report that products on the shelf at a big chain store were missing a key ingredient: Aloe Vera. So stay with quality brands. One study found di(2-ethyl-hexyl) phthalate (DEHP) in Aloe vera which inhibited growth of three leukemia cell lines and reduced AF-2-induced mutagenicity. Another study showed that Acemannan stimulates the immune system production of IL-6 and TNF-α and nitric oxide release which could be responsible for some of its anticancer powers. Another study verified that Aloeride is a new immunostimulatory polysaccharide found in commercial Aloe vera juice. Another study confirmed that Aloe-emodin has antiproliferative and pro-apoptotic effects against two human liver cancer cell lines. Another study showed that the percentage of both tumor regression and disease control was significantly higher in patients treated with Aloe while on chemotherapy. A study showed that Aloe has antigenotoxic potential and noted a potential use in the prevention of DNA damage caused by known chemical mutagens.[33]

10. AMARANTH (Amaranthus viridis)

Top Recommended Edible Plant: Seeds are used to make flour and young shoots and leaves are used like Spinach. Amaranth has a long list of holistic medicinal properties too. One study showed that all extracts displayed antiproliferative activity against Jurkat, CEM, and HL-60. Another study showed that extracts had significant anticancer effects on HT-29 and HepG2 cells. Another study showed significant inhibition of HT-29 cell growth.[34]

11. AMLA (Phyllanthus emblica)

Top Recommended Edible Fruit: Part of the Ayurvedic medicine of ancient India in a formula called Triphala, which is considered one of their most potent medicines, Amla and Triphala are both suspected to have anticancer power. Incidentally, Black Myrobalan and another species of Terminalia (T. belerica) are the other fruits used in Triphala and Black Myrobalan is also in this list.[34]

12. ANDROGRAPHIS (Andrographis paniculata) *IM

Top Recommended Holistic Herb: This plant has gotten a lot of hype recently, but it is well deserved. One study showed that the antioxidant action of the aqueous extract may play a role in its anticarcinogenic activity. Another study showed the activity of an extract against the HEP2 cell line. [36]

13. ANGELICA (Angelica archangelica)

Top Recommended Holistic Herb: This close relative to celery has at least one thing in common with its culinary sister: it is loaded with phytoestrogens and has a long history of usage in female hormonal health issues. Some phytoestrogens have been found to be potent cancer fighting compounds as well. Because Angelica is potent medicine, moderation is advised.[40]

14. ANISE (Pimpinella anisum)

Top Recommended Culinary Spice: Although Star-Anise is a different species, the two are interchangeable and have very similar biochemistry. Anise, yet another relative of celery, is also loaded with phytoestrogen, in this case Anethole. Phytoestrogens have been linked to alleviating women's hormonal issues, but they have also been found to have cancer fighting properties as well. Because Anise has a very high Anethole content, moderation is advised.[41]

15. ANNATTO (Bixa orellana)

Top Recommended Culinary Herb: The brick red seeds of the "Lipstick Tree" contain Bixin, a unique phytonutrient, and add a beautiful golden color and earthy flavor to soups and stews. But overindulgence is not recommended. Adding a pinch now and again can be very beneficial to your health. One study showed cytotoxicity against B16F10 cells. Analysis found three known anticancer compounds: Geranyl Geraniol, Squalene, and beta-Sitosterol. [42]

16. ANT PLANT (Hydnophytum formicarum)

A flavonoid derivative, 7,3',5'-trihydroxyflavanone (3HFD) isolated from H. formicarum has shown cytotoxic effects on the MCF-7 cell line by inducing apoptosis. [43]

17. APPLE (Malus domestica)

Top Recommended Edible Fruit: Apples contain many active compounds including Quercetin which is a powerful antioxidant phenolic compound that has been well studied and has shown tremendous health benefits including: lowering the risk of various forms of cancer, halting the growth of breast, colon, prostate, endometrial and lung cancers, lowers blood pressure, lowers several risk factors of heart disease, and lowers cholesterol.[490]

18. APRICOT (Prunus armeniaca)

Top Recommended Edible Fruit: Apricots are loaded with some powerful phytonutrients including: Quercetin, Anthocyanidins and Catechins which have studies showing anticancer powers.[491]

19. AQUATIC ROTULA (Rotula aquatica)

Recommended Holistic Herb: One study isolated polyphenols with strong antioxidant activity suggesting the herb could be used as protection for patients undergoing radiation therapy. Another study showed an extract had extremely effective antiproliferative action against a pancreatic cancer cell line. [48]

20. ARTILLERY PLANT (Pilea microphylla)

Recommended Holistic Herb: Often called "Artillery Fern" this small soft fleshy herb is actually a flowering plant although the tiny green flowers often go unnoticed. One study showed that that the polyphenols present in the extract provided protection of V79 cells from Gamma radiation injury. Alone, the study wouldn't say much, but some plants have been shown to have radioprotective power against solar short-wave UV and Gamma radiation exposure and this is a RARE and valuable property.[49]

21. ARUGULA (Eruca sativa)

Top Recommended Edible Plant: Its greatest health benefits come from the Isothiocyanates – sulfur-containing compounds that are potent antioxidants. These phytonutrients in Arugula have been shown to: reduce the risk of cancer and actively combat existing cancer. [492]

22. ASHITABA (Angelica keiskei)

Top Recommended Edible Holistic Herb: Ashitaba has a long list of holistic medicinal properties, but make absolutely certain that you are getting the real plant and not a cheap (and ineffective) substitute. A study showed a chalconoid in the plant can inhibit the proliferation of hepatocarcinoma cells in vivo. A study of the stems found Xanthoangelol and 4-Hydroxyderricin. These chalcanoids showed growth inhibition of KATO III cells via apoptosis.[52]

23. ASOKA TREE (Saraca indica)

Asoka Tree bark extract showed significant inhibition of the HeLa cell line. Another study isolated a new diterpenoid: 6,9-epoxy Marrubiinic Acid, which showed cytotoxicity against human cancer cell lines. Another study showed antimutagenic activity and antigenotoxic properties against cyclophosphamide, a known toxin that damages DNA. [53]

24. ASPARAGUS (Asparagus spp.)

Top Recommended Edible Plant: Asparagus has a lot going for it; it's nutritious, loaded with antioxidants and may fight cancer too. One study of the roots yielded a new and unique phytosterol, Sarsasapogenin O, which showed significant cytotoxicity against human A2780, HO-8910, Eca-109, MGC-803, CNE, LTEP-a-2, and KB tumor cells. Asparaginase, a main compound in the plant, has been reported to have curative potential versus cancer. A study showed that the saponins in Asparagus inhibited the growth of HepG2. [25]

25. ASTRAGALUS (Astragalus membranaceus) *IM

Top Recommended Holistic Herb: Astragalus is one of the legendary components of Traditional Chinese Medicine and it is a well known immunostimulant that can help folks recover quickly from chemotherapy treatments. One study has shown that it also has direct anticancer properties inducing cell death in at least one form of leukemia.[55]

26. AVOCADO (Persea americana)

Top Recommended Edible Fruit: Avocado contains a special group of monounsaturated fatty acids that have been shown to have significant health benefits including anti-inflammatory, hypolipidemic and hypotensive properties. Avocados are rich in Vitamin B9 – Folate and Fiber as well as Potassium. A study of three biologically active compounds in the unripe fruit showed activity against six human cancer cell lines with selectivity against human prostate adenocarcinoma. Another study isolated a Persealide (compounds unique to Avocados) which showed cytotoxicity against three cancers: human lung, breast and colon carcinomas.[411]

27. BAEL (Aegle marmelos)

Top Recommended Edible Fruit: Bael is a bit unusual looking inside but it brings a lot of powerful nutrients. One study showed protection against Doxorubicin-induced genotoxicity in mice bone marrow. Another study found 1,2,3-Propanetriol as the major component of the leaf extract followed by Cinnamic Acid Methyl Ester, 3,4-dihydro-4,5-dihydroxy-1(2H)-Naphthalenone, Phytol, and Nicotinamide. The extract induced apoptosis in HepG2. [58]

28. BAMBOO ORCHID (Arundina graminifolia)

Many species of Orchids, Lilies and grasses are toxic, but many others are not, namely; Barley (an edible grass,) Garlic (an edible lily rhizome,) and Vanilla (an edible Orchid seed pod.) A study of Bamboo Orchid found 11 new compounds. Some of these showed significant cytotoxicity against five cancer cell lines. Another study evaluated Gramniphenol H and I. "H" showed cytotoxicity on PC3 cells, while "I" showed cytotoxicity against NB4 and PC3 cells. A study isolated other compounds and found significant anti-tumor activity. Another study discovered two new stilbenoids: Arundinan and Arundinaol and showed they possessed strong anti-tumor activity in vitro. Another study isolated a new flavonoid: 3(S),4(S)-3',4'-dihydroxyl-7,8,-methylene-dioxyl-pterocarpan which showed high cytotoxicity on the SH-SY5Y cell line. [59]

29. BANDICOOT BERRY (Leea indica)

A study showed that a fraction had significant cytotoxicity against CaSki cells by growth suppression and apoptosis. Another study showed a crude extract of the leaves had significant anti-tumor, antioxidant, and cytotoxic activity on EAC cells in vivo. A study of leaf extracts showed selective in vitro cytotoxicity against DU-145 and PC-3 cell lines.[61]

30. BARBERRY (Berberis vulgaris)

Top Recommended Holistic Herb: Forget the berries; it is the bark of the plant that is used. It contains the alkaloids: Berberine, Oxyacanthine, and Columbamine. Berberine has well documented scientific evidence showing it is a potent COX-2 inhibitor which makes it a powerful anti-inflammatory and anti-tumor agent. But moderation is advised; Barberry can have negative effects on the heart.[63]

31. BASIL (Ocimum basilicum)

Top Recommended Culinary Spice: There are many dozens of cultivated varieties of Basil but simple dried leaf Basil found in the grocery store spice section is good enough and brings plenty of powerful holistic medicinal benefits. Add it to soups, stews, salads, casseroles, home made Oil and Vinegar dressing or even herbal teas to get in on the amazing power of this Top Recommended Spice. A study showed Sweet Basil oil had marked antiproliferative activity on KB and P388 cell lines. [66]

32. BAYUR (Pterospermum acerifolium)
One study showed that fractions of leaves, flowers, and bark all had effective antioxidant and DNA protection activity.[67]

33. BEET (Beta vulgaris)
Top Recommended Edible Plant: Beets are very low calorie and contain a whole group of unique phytochemicals called Betalains that are the subject of current intense scientific investigation for their potential health benefits. Raw Beet Root juice is already considered to have extraordinary medicinal power. One study compared red beetroot extract with the chemotherapy drug Doxorubicin on human prostate and human breast cancer cells and showed Betanin, the major betacyanin constituent, may play a role in the comparable anticancer power of the extract.[26][493]

34. BENGAL DAYFLOWER (Commelina benghalensis)
A study showed that an extract contains compounds that may be beneficial against malignant tumors. Another study showed it has antiproliferative properties vs Wil-2NS.[68]

35. BERMUDA GRASS (Cynodon dactylon)
Top Recommended Edible Plant: I bet you never thought you would eat grass! Well, it's more of an herbal tea which can be prepared from all parts of the plant and it has a very long list of holistic medicinal properties, but make absolutely certain that you have the correct species. One study showed activity against EAC in vivo. Another study showed activity against HEP-2. Another study showed an extract of the roots had liver protective activity against DEN-induced liver cancer in vivo. Another in vivo study of an extract of the leaves showed significant anti-tumor activity versus EAC and a significant hepatoprotective effect. [70]

36. BETEL PEPPER (Piper betle)
Top Recommended Culinary Spice: This spice has potent health benefits just like its far more common relative Black Pepper (P. nigrum.) One study showed that an extract administered ½ hour prior to exposure provided protection against Gamma radiation and Cyclophosphamide. Another study showed that an extract of the leaves has significant cytotoxicity against the Hep-2 cell line. Another study of leaf extracts showed tumor inhibition of human melanoma in vivo. Another study showed an extract of the leaves had anti-tumor activity against EAC in vivo. Another study showed that oral feeding of P. betle leaf extract significantly inhibited the growth of human prostate xenografts in vivo. The study isolated Hydroxychavicol (HC) and Chavibetol (CHV) and found HC to be eight times more potent than CHV.[72]

37. BIGNAY (Antidesma bunius)
Top Recommended Edible Fruit: Bignay is native to Australia

and the surrounding regions and is very tart, but it has some exceptional phytonutrients. A study of the polyphenol content of Bignay dried leaf extract showed tumor inhibiting antiangiogenic activity. [73]

38. BIRCH (Betula alba)

Top Recommended Holistic Herb: Birch bark and leaf herbal tea contains Betulins and Betulinic Acid which have been shown to have anticancer properties.[75]

39. BITTER MELON (Momordica charantia)

Top Recommended Edible Fruit: Bitter melon does have a few cases of poisoning from it likely due to overindulgence and eating the unripe melons. However, it has several studies indicating anticancer effects. In one study its antioxidants were shown to help prevent damage from well known carcinogens. In another, it specifically prevented carcinogens from causing breast cancer. In another study it prevented DNA damage to colon cells. Another three independent studies showed significant chemoprotective and antimutagenic power. Another study showed that M. charantia induced cell death in nasopharyngeal carcinoma cells. Another study isolated 19 unique cucurbitacins: Kuguacin A to S. Kuguacin J decreased LNCaP cell proliferation and viability. Another study showed that the aqueous extract induced cell death in six different cancer cell lines.[76]

40. BLACK CURRANT (Antidesma ghaesembilla)

Top Recommended Edible Fruit: Black currents are loaded with Vitamin C and antioxidants and one study isolated Vomifoliol from the leaves. Naturally occurring compounds similar to this one have been found to have antiproliferative and cytotoxic effects against cancer cells.[77]

41. BLACK MYROBALAN (Terminalia chebula) *IM

Top Recommended Holistic Herb: "Ink Nut" as it is also called is another ingredient in the legendary Triphala medicine of ancient India and it has an impressive list of medicinal properties and many of them have been verified in scientific studies. A study showed anticancer effects of an aqueous extract on A549.[78]

42. BLACK PEPPER (Piper nigrum)

Top Recommended Culinary Spice: Black pepper is the second most heavily traded spice on Earth after salt. But while salt may be a necessary evil (we do need the Sodium, Chlorine and Iodine it provides) it is fair to say that Black Pepper is far better for human health and studies have verified a long list of benefits including its ability to aid digestion and may help prevent and fight certain types of colon cancer. With an impressive ORAC Score of 34,053 and a highly volatile active component named Piperine (it gives pepper its distinctive aroma, flavor, and tendency to make you sneeze) it is best to apply it from a fresh peppercorn grinder after you remove the food from the heat. One study showed that black pepper has a strong immunomodulatory action that may help prevent cancer.

Other studies have shown that Piperine selectively targets and kills certain colon cancer cell lines while promoting the production of digestive enzymes and the break down of fats and helping healthy intestinal cells absorb nutrients.[450]

43. BLESSED THISTLE (Cnicus benedictus)
Top Recommended Holistic Herb: Well known as a depurative that promotes both diuresis and diaphoresis, Blessed Thistle is also a powerful liver detoxifier and it contains phytoestrogens that are effective in helping women's hormonal issues as well. At least one study has shown that it has potent anti-tumor and anticancer properties. [451]

44. BLUEBERRY (Vaccinium corymbosa)
Top Recommended Edible Fruit: Blueberries are showing up at the top of lists like "Foods you should never eat" but that is due to pesticide contamination and MOST organic products are clean. Blueberries contain high amounts of anthocyanidins as well as Pterostilbene. Studies have shown that Pterostilbene is a powerful anti-inflammatory, antioxidant, neuroprotective, antimutagen and reduces the risk of cancer, and halts the growth of many forms of cancer.[494]

45. BLUMEA (Blumea lacera)
There are two species of Blumea in this list which tells the story that these plants have powerful phytonutrients and antioxidants that promote health. One study of Bangladeshi medicinal plants showed an extract had the highest cytotoxicity against human gastric, colon, and breast cancer cell lines.[452]

46. BLUMEA CAMPHOR (Blumea balsamifera)
Two studies of extracts showed selective growth inhibition in hepatocellular carcinoma cells and no cytotoxicity toward normal hepatocytes in vivo. Another study of leaf extract yielded nine flavonoids. Some showed anti-tyrosinase activity (an anticancer property) stronger than Arbutin. Others showed cytotoxicity against KB and human lung cancer cell lines.[453]

47. BOK CHOY (Brassica rapa)
Top Recommended Edible Plant: Glucosinolates are sulfur containing organic compounds found in high abundance in plants belonging to the Brassicaceae family. One study showed that the glucosinolates in the crude extract provide potent antimutagenic protection for human lymphocytes.[28]

48. BONESET (Eupatorium perfoliatum) *IM
Top Recommended Holistic Herb: Its name comes from its ability to treat "Bonebreak fever" a.k.a. Dengue fever. Boneset is a depurative through diuresis and diaphoresis and it is also known to be a potent immunostimulant and will serve as an excellent tonic to help recover from chemotherapy treatments. It also contains many flavonoids including: Quercetin, Kaempferol, Rutin and Eupatorin which have all been shown to have direct anticancer properties. Boneset tea is also called Oswego Tea.[79]

49. BORAGE (Borago officinalis) *IM
Top Recommended Holistic Herb: Loaded with Gamma-Linoleic Acid which has been shown to have anti-tumor effects against certain breast cancer cell lines, it also boosts the immune system and that is our first line of defense against all disease including cancer.[80]

50. BOTTLE GOURD (Lagenaria siceraria)
Be aware that there are rare reports of toxicity likely caused by either extreme overindulgence or an allergic reaction. A study showed an extract of the fruit possessed antimutagenic properties. Another study of the fruit showed significant reduction of DNA damage induced by Cyclophosphamide in bone marrow cells. Another study of an extract showed strong inhibition of cancer cell growth of the A549 cell line.[83]

51. BREADFRUIT (Artocarpus altilis)
Top Recommended Edible Fruit: The fruit is usually cooked because it is starchy. However, it does have nutritional value and is a main staple for many small tropical island nations. A study evaluated the wood extract on the T47D cell line and showed decreased cell viability.[85]

52. BROCCOLI (Brassica oleracea)
Top Recommended Superfood: Broccoli is an excellent source of Chromium; about two cups provides you with 100% RDA of this critical mineral that is very difficult to find in sufficient quantities in most foods. It is also very low calorie and has chlorophylls which help detoxify the liver. Studies have shown decreased mortality rates in radiation-exposed lab animals fed broccoli and cabbage. Some isothiocyanates, found in Brassicas, have been shown to inhibit tumors induced by chemical carcinogens. Indole-3-carbinol showed anticarcinogenesis effects in vivo. Sulforaphane inhibits H. pylori (bacteria that can cause ulcers and stomach cancer) and prevents Benzo-a-pyrene-induced stomach tumors. Cancer cells containing Bcl-2 have increased resistance to chemotherapy but one study showed that Bcl-2 cannot protect cancer cells against isothiocyanates in natural foods. Another study showed that the compounds found in the cruciferous vegetables block human lung cancer cell progression both in vivo and in vitro.[8]

53. BUCKWHEAT (Fagopyrum esculentum)
Top Recommended Cereal: Buckwheat isn't a grain; it's a seed. Nevertheless it is classified as a grain. Aside from being high in Manganese, Copper, Magnesium, Phosphorus, and Fiber studies have shown that the Lignans in Buckwheat are converted by the intestinal bacteria into "mammalian lignans" which protect the body against hormone-dependent forms of cancer including breast cancer.[489]

54. BULL'S HEART (Annona reticulata)
Top Recommended Edible Fruit: Leaves can also be made into herbal tea fresh or dried. This is one of over 160 species of the

Annona genus almost all of which produce edible fruit. A. reticulata is not as well known as Custard Apple (A. squamosa) or Soursop (A. muricata) both of which are also Top recommended Edible Fruits and herbal tea leaves in this list. A study of Annonacin isolated from the seeds showed it caused significant cell death in various cancer lines. Another study showed a root extract to have significant antiproliferative activity against A549, K562, HeLa and MDA-MB human cancer cell lines. Another study showed a leaf extract had anticancer power against HCT15, Hop65, and HepG2 cancer cell lines attributed to acetogenins.[86]

55. BURDOCK (Arctium lappa)
Top Recommended Edible/Holistic Herb: Burdock root is used in some Japanese dishes and is very rich in potassium and contains Arctigenin (a phytoestrogen.) In one study this was shown to induce apoptosis in lung adenocarcinoma cells.[87]

56. BURI PALM (Corypha utan)
Piceantannol, a stilbenoid, isolated from the seeds showed very strong cytotoxic activity against P388 cells.[88]

57. BURR MARIGOLD (Bidens pilosa)
Burr marigold is one of the most widespread invasive weeds on Earth. I have a large stand of them in my own yard and they spread like crazy. However, overindulgence has been linked to mutagenicity. An irony considering that the young shoots and leaves are edible and it has a long list of beneficial properties including some studies showing it to have anticancer powers.[89]

58. BUSH MINT (Hyptis suaveolens)
Recommended Holistic Herb: This is another relatively rare herb that may be difficult to locate and be wary of substitutions. One study showed potent cytotoxicity against EAC via apoptosis.[90]

59. BUTTERNUT SQUASH (Cucurbita moschata)
Top Recommended Edible Fruit: Many members of the Cucurbit family (Cucumbers and their kin) are considered "vegetables" not fruit, but no matter what you decide to call them, they all contain Cucurbitacins which have been shown in numerous studies to actively combat cancer. Butternut squash has a unique protein that studies have shown halts the growth of certain forms of melanoma skin cancer.[495]

60. BUTTON MUSHROOM (Agaricus bisporus) *IM
Top Recommended Edible Mushroom: It's all about the beta-Glucans. These unusual polysaccharides found in mushrooms (and Oats and Barley) have been shown in numerous recent studies to have powerful immunostimulant and anticancer activity. While the other edible mushrooms in this list are expensive gourmet mushrooms and have much higher concentrations of the almighty beta-Glucans, plain white Button Mushrooms found in your local grocery store are related to Agaricus blazei which costs plenty more, and both the Button and the Portabella (varieties of

the same species) have beta-Glucans in them too, but at a fraction of the price.[30][74][332]

61. CABBAGE (Brassica oleracea)

Top Recommended Superfood: Why is Cabbage a superfood? 1) Very low calorie, 2) Higher in Vitamin C by weight, amt/cal and amt/cost than Grapefruit, and 3) It contains glucosinolates which are of enormous interest to medical science. A study found that cabbage is a good source of antioxidant and anti-inflammatory compounds for the prevention of chronic disease associated with oxidative stress such as cancer and heart disease. It contains Indole-3-carbinol, Glucobrassicin and Sinigrin. It is known that the body converts these into other forms that have proven anticancer properties. A study evaluated 2-Pyrrolidinone for antioxidant and anticancer activity and it showed cytotoxicity on HeLa and PC-3 cell lines. Another study tested the glucosinolates and other compounds and showed that Cabbage has antioxidant activity up to five times greater than Vitamin C alone. [4]

62. CACAO (Theobroma cacao)

Top Recommended Superfood: Every time I suggest to people that Dark Chocolate is not just delicious, but also a Superfood, they think I am insane. Four ounces of Pure 100% Cacao brings 100% RDA of both Iron and Magnesium, both of which are very difficult to get in sufficient amounts from any other food source on a daily basis. Add to that its antioxidant score of 49,944 (the highest ORAC score of any edible food excluding spices) and additional potential holistic health benefits and you must concede that 100% pure unsweetened Baker's Dark Chocolate may be one of the few true miracle foods on Earth. Several studies concluded that dietary polyphenols, in large amounts, can exert a desirable effect on certain forms of cancer. Its main flavonoids are Flavan-3-ols; Epicatechin and Catechin both of which are well known for their anticancer power. In vivo studies showed the antiproliferative effect of a cocoa-rich diet. In vitro studies showed inhibitory effect on CaCo-2 through non-apoptotic cell death. A review lists the phenolic compounds found in Cacao and the promising effects on the cancer cell lines tested: polymer procyanidins vs. Caco-2; Procyanidin B2 vs. Caco-2 and HL-60; Epicatechin vs. Caco-2, SH-SY5Y, HepG3, and MCF-7; 3'-O-methyl epicatechin vs. FEK4; and Catechin vs. HepG2, Caco-2, and Int-407. Another study showed fractions of cacao seed had anti-tumor activity on the L5178Y cell line.[12]

63. CAESAR WEED (Urena lobata)

A study of extracts of the plant showed significant antiproliferative and antioxidant properties against the MDA-MB-435 cell line.[91]

64. CALABASH TREE (Crescentia cujete)

A study of Calabash fruit showed antiangiogenic effect that has potential for halting tumor growth.[92]

65. CANISTEL (Pouteria campechiana)

Top Recommended Edible Fruit: This fruit tree belongs to another vast genus of tropical fruiting trees most of which are edible and highly prized in their native ranges. Canistel, more commonly called "Eggfruit" is one of the smaller fruits, about twice the size of an egg, egg-shaped and bright yellow. But the tree is one of the taller ones in a genus of big trees reaching 70 feet in ideal native Southeast Asian Rain Forest habitats. One study of the leaf extracts showed the antimutagenic activity of Canistel.[93]

66. CANNA LILY (Canna indica)

Edible rhizomes: Canna is a large perennial lily to over 6 feet tall in a spreading rosette of huge broadsword-shaped leaves and a central stem topped in large red flowers and is very popular in commercial landscaping. But the young tubers are edible and the plant is highly prized in its native ranges. One study yielded: Stigmasterol and 6-beta-hydroxystigmasta-4, 22-diene-3-one, both already known to have anticancer properties.[94]

67. CANNONBALL TREE (Couroupita guianensis)

These large odd fruits are rarely eaten because of their offensive odor, but they do pack a punch. Isatin (1H-indole-2,3-dione) has been isolated from the flowers and the derivatives are known to be cytotoxic to human carcinoma cell lines.[95]

68. CANTALOUPE (Cucumis melo)

Top Recommended Edible Fruit: Cantaloupes are widely available, delicious and bring nutrition as well as health benefits. One study of the stems isolated 21 cucurbitacins including 9 new ones. Cucurbitacin A and B showed significant cytotoxicity and antiproliferation of A549/ATCC and BEL7402 cells. Cucurbitacins are triterpenoids, predominantly found in the Cucurbitaceae family (Cucumbers and their kin.) A study of an aqueous extract of the fruit pulp showed significant antioxidant power against hydroxyl, superoxide, and nitric oxide radicals and was found to be cytotoxic against EAC cells. Another study showed significant anti-tumor effects both in vivo and in vitro. Another study of the aqueous fruit extract showed cytotoxicity against the PC-3 cell line. A study of an extract showed reduction of BPH with apoptotic activity both in vitro and in vivo. A study of an aqueous seed extract showed cytotoxic effects against EAC cells. Another study of an extract showed strong toxicity against A375 cancer cells. Cucumbers and all of their kin should be featured in any diet for the prevention and treatment of cancer.[31]

69. CAPE GOOSEBERRY (Physalis peruviana)

Top Recommended Edible Fruit: Physalis is a vast genus with many small edible berries that are closely related to tomatoes. They are powerful medicine and overindulgence of any species is not recommended. One study showed the extract induced HepG2 apoptosis. Another study isolated 4beta-Hydroxy-withanolide from Cape Gooseberries and showed it had anticancer potency against H1299. Another study showed antioxidant and cytotoxic activities of edible parts of P. peruviana on the HT-29, Hep3B, SaOS-2, and SH-SY5Y cell lines. Cape gooseberries are effective against a wide range of cancers.[96]

70. CAPER THORN (Capparis micracantha)

A study of an extract of the leaves showed inhibitory effect against a form of lung cancer. [97]

71. CARABAO'S TEATS (Uvaria rufa)

A study yielded one new lignan glycoside, Ufaside, along with six known compounds: Oxoanolobine, Ergosta-4,6,8(14),22-tetraen-3-one, Catechin, Epicatechin, Daucosterol, and Glutin-5-en-3-one. Compounds 2 and 3 showed cytotoxicity against the LU-1 cell line.[98]

72. CARAWAY (Carum carvi)

Top Recommended Culinary Spice: Although the seeds have a strong licorice-like flavor and are commonly used in Rye Bread crust, the roots, stalks, leaves, etc. are all edible. No surprise since the plant is a close relative to carrots and celery. It is the Carvone and Limonene content, both strong monoterpenoids that have been shown in studies to have many health benefits including anticancer potential.[99]

73. CARDAMOM (Elettaria cardamomum)

Top Recommended Culinary Spice: This close relative to ginger is loaded with Terpene, Terpineol, and Cineol, simple terpenoids that pack a powerful punch that might help fight cancer.[100]

74. CARIBBEAN SLASH PINE (Pinus caribaea)

A study showed extracts have antimutagenic components other than its antioxidants. Another study showed the procyanidins from the bark have strong antioxidant and inhibitory activity on HL-60 cells, and effective inhibitory activity against the BGC-823, and BEL-7402 cell lines.[101]

75. CARPETWEED (Mollugo pentaphylla)

A study showed anti-tumor activity against implanted malignant tumors and promoted significant recovery of leukocytes from radiation damage.[102]

76. CARROT (Daucus carota)

Top Recommended Superfood: Carrots are simply too good to ignore. One medium sized carrot brings about 200% RDA of Vitamin A as beta-Carotene which is also a powerful antioxidant. One study of the seed extract showed it inhibited the growth of EAC in vivo. Aqueous extract showed relatively high antioxidant activity and suppressed tumor production in skin. Another study showed the anticancer effect of fractions of the oil extract on the MDA-MB-231 and MCF-7 cell lines. Another study of the oil extract showed a significant increase in cell death and decrease in cell proliferation against four human cancer cell lines: HT-29, CaCo-2, MCF-7, and MDA-MB-231. A study of carrot juice extract showed apoptosis on both myeloid and lymphoid leukemia cell lines.[5]

77. CASHEW (Anacardium occidentale)

Top Recommended Edible Fruit/Nut: Most people appreciate the Cashew nut, but few are aware that the fruit is also quite edible as well. Overindulgence is not recommended as it can become toxic in excess and Cashew is also a known allergen. Cashew gum polysaccharide, with branched b-Galactose and other oligosaccharides and proteins showed high inhibitory activity against an implanted S-180 solid tumor in vivo. A study of the leaf extract was cytotoxic and pro-apoptotic on lymphoblast leukemia cells. [32]

78. CELANDINE (Chelidonium majus) *IM

Top Recommended Holistic Herb: The studies are limited as to its anticancer properties, but it contains: Berberine, Sanguinarine, Chelidonine, Protopine, Coptisine, and Stylopine. Berberine has many studies showing that it does have anticancer properties and Sanguinarine has at least one study showing possible potent anticancer activity as well. The plant with the highest concentration is called Bloodroot which happens to be quite toxic but Celandine is much safer and is often used as an herbal tea with depurative power and as a helper for the gall bladder and bile issues.[103]

79. CELERY (Apium graveolens)

Top Recommended Culinary Spice/Edible Plant: The seeds are a spice and the stalks are an excellent appetizer or addition to salads, soups, stews, and casseroles. Celery is one of my top recommended "Net Negative Calorie" foods meaning it has extremely low calories but it also possesses some very potent phytonutrients too. Celery is a member of an enormous family of plants all of which are loaded with phytoestrogens. Celery has large quantities of both Apiole and Apigenin. One study showed a seed extract was antiproliferative in vitro on DAL and L929. [24]

80. CEYLON BOX WOOD (Psydrax dicoccos)

A study of an extract of the leaf yielded: Caryophyllene oxide, Spathulenol, Cedren-13-ol, Ledene oxide, m-mentho-4,8-diene and 2-Furancarboxaldehyde. Some of these constituents are similar to compounds known to have immunomodulatory, anti-tumor, and antioxidant properties. [104]

81. CHAFF FLOWER (Achyranthes aspera)

Top Recommended Edible Plant: Leaves and seeds are edible with very low toxicity detected. Studies have shown anticancer activity on several different cancer types including a form of pancreatic cancer. A study showed significant inhibition of EBV-EA induced by Raji cancer cells. A study of a leaf extract showed cytotoxicity on several tumor cell lines, with the pancreatic cells showing the most sensitivity. Another study showed anticancer effects in vivo. This is one of VERY FEW plants that has shown remarkable evidence of action against forms of pancreatic cancer – one of the deadliest kinds of cancer.[105]

82. CHAGA MUSHROOM (Inonotus obliquus) *IM

Top Recommended Edible Mushroom: Chaga or Cinder Conk

belongs to a group of parasitic fungi that kill trees and it has a long medicinal history in Siberia and North America for longevity and health tonics. Chaga is usually taken as a medicinal tea and other supplement products are available. The active compounds in edible mushrooms (many featured in this list) are beta-Glucans which have numerous studies showing that they are powerful immunostimulants and anti-tumor agents.[74][106][332]

83. CHAMBER BITTER (Phyllanthus urinaria)

Recommended Holistic Herb: Better known for its benefits to the kidney and bladder and its folkloric usage to help break up kidney stones, the plant has some unique and potentially very effective pathways to defeating cancer cells called telomerase inhibition. One study investigated the effect of P urinaria on telomerase activity and apoptosis in NPC-BM1 cells and found: Gallic Acid, Brevifolin Carboxylic Acid, Corilagin, Phyllanthusiin C and Ellagic Acid as possible causes of the effect. A study showed the aqueous extract induced apoptosis in HL-60. Another study suggests the anticancer power is mainly due to induced apoptosis of cancer cells through DNA fragmentation possibly caused by telomerase activity. Another study showed inhibition of 143B cell growth via apoptosis. Effective treatments of bone cancers like this one are EXCEEDINGLY RARE.[107]

84. CHANCA PIEDRA (Phyllanthus niruri) *IM

Top Recommended Holistic Herb: Where to begin with this one? Chanca Piedra has been studied primarily for its reputation for breaking up kidney and gallstones and this has been confirmed. Chanca Piedra is nephroprotective, but it is also hepatoprotective, hypoglycemic, hypolipidemic and hypotensive. Finally, there are preliminary studies showing that it has significant anticancer power as well. Studies have shown efficacy against skin carcinogenesis, MCF-7, A549, COR-L23, MOLT4, and K562 cell lines. Verify the species and use in moderation; there is not enough information concerning chronic toxicity. [108]

85. CHAYOTE (Sechium edule)

Top Recommended Edible Plant: This is another member of the amazing Cucurbit family. While the Chayote squash is usually what consumers find in the fresh produce section of their grocery store, all parts of the plant are edible from the roots to the stems, leaves and fruit. One study showed the antiproliferative activity of crude fruit extracts against all HeLa tumor cell lines tested.[109]

86. CHERIMOYA (Annona cherimola)

Top Recommended Edible Fruit: Cherimoya is a member of a genus of over 160 species of edible fruit trees that most folks have never heard of before. Most of the fruits of the genus are large and Cherimoya is no exception weighing several pounds each and while most Annona species fruits are quite sweet and delicious, those familiar with them consider Cherimoya to be the best and deserving of consideration as the best tasting fruit on Earth. A new compound was found in the seeds: Cherimolacyclopeptide C which showed significant cytotoxicity in vitro against the KB cell line.[110]

87. CHICKENWEED (Portulaca quadrifida)

All species of Portulaca are edible (leaves and soft stems) raw or cooked, but only in limited amounts. A study of the extracts of P. quadrifida showed significant and selective effect against HT-29 cells with less activity against normal colon cells.[111]

88. CHICO SAPODILLA (Manilkara zapota)

Top Recommended Edible Fruit: A distant relative to Sapodilla whose roots were once used to make root beer, it should come as no surprise that the fruits taste like pears dipped in root beer and are very sweet. A study of the stem bark showed significant anti-tumor activity against EAC in vivo. Another study showed that a fruit extract was cytotoxic toward several cancer cell lines.[112]

89. CHICORY (Cichorium intybus) *IM

Top Recommended Edible Plant: Chicory has a long usage as a coffee substitute, but it contains Inulin, Cichoriin, Taraxasterol, Tannins, Pectin, and Esculetin. It is a powerful anti-inflammatory and immunostimulant which can help patients recover from chemotherapy. Also, some of those compounds have been found to have anticancer activity.[113]

90. CHINA ROSE HIBISCUS (Hibiscus rosa-sinensis)

Recommended Holistic Herb: There are several species of Hibiscus in this list. Be sure not to overindulge as it can become toxic. One study showed the extract has an inhibitory effect on the tumor promotion stage of skin cancer. Hibiscus tea is normally prescribed to lower blood pressure, and it is very effective but it is also very powerful medicine: moderation is advised.[114]

91. CHINESE BELL FLOWER (Abutilon indicum) *IM

A study showed fractions of A. indicum leaves had considerable cytotoxicity on U87MG cells. [115]

92. CHINESE BURR (Triumfetta bartramia)

A study of an extract showed significant anti-tumor effects against DAL in vivo.[116]

93. CHINESE CROTON (Excoecaria cochinchinensis)

One study of extracts from 29 Indonesian plants tested in vitro against human lung, colon and stomach cancer cells; found that the extracts showed powerful selective cytotoxicity toward various cancer cell lines.[117]

94. CHINESE JUNIPER (Juniperus chinensis)

A study showed significant anti-metastatic effect of an extract on 26-M3.1 cells. Another study showed cytotoxic and apoptotic activity of the phytochemical Widdrol extracted from J. chinensis against the HT29 cell line. [118]

95. CHINESE LANTERN (Physalis angulata)

Top Recommended Edible Fruit: There are many species of Physalis and most are relatively small plants that yield edible fruits.

Proper identification of the species is a must, since many resemble each other though none are truly dangerous. But overindulgence is not recommended because they contain powerful phytochemicals. A study showed antiproliferative and apoptotic effects on MDA-MB 231 and MCF-7 cell lines. Another study showed that fruit capsule fractions had significant cancer inhibition effects. Physalin F has shown anti-tumor activity against five human cancer lines, the most potent activity was on HA22T. Another study isolated three withanolides and showed Physangulidine-A significantly reduced two hormone-independent prostate cancer cell lines via antimitotic and apoptotic effects. A study of extracts showed anti-metastatic and antiangiogenic activity against HSC-3 and human umbilical vein endothelial cells. Another study showed cytotoxic effects towards: HeLa, KB, Colo 205, Calu and MCF-7 cells in vitro. A study isolated a new withanolide, Physaguilide P, which showed significant cytotoxicity against MG-63, HepG2 and MDA-MB-231. Another study showed Physalin B was cytotoxic towards A375 and A2058 cells and noted Physalin B induces apoptosis of malignant melanoma cancer cells. [119]

96. CHINESE LANTERN TREE (Hernandia guianensis)

This plant contains a precursor to a recognized anticancer drug and has shown in several studies to have potent anticancer power, but there is little information regarding its safety and caution is advised. One study isolated an alkaloid with inhibitory activity against Walker 256. Another study reports the seeds contain 2.4% Deoxypodophyllotoxin which is a form of Epipodophyllotoxin, a basic skeleton of the anticancer drug Etoposide. Another study reported Thalicarpine, isolated from the stem-bark, has tumor inhibitory power. A 1975 study isolated eight compounds: Desoxypodophyllotoxin, Dehydrothalicarpine, Thalicarpine, Ovigerine, Hernangerine, Hernandonine and two unidentified compounds. Desoxypodophyllotoxin and Thalicarpine showed cytotoxicity on nasopharyngeal carcinoma. Another study isolated seven lignans and all inhibited EBV-EA in Raji cancer cells. [120]

97. CHINESE PERFUME PLANT (Aglaia odorata)

A study isolated Rocaglaol which showed distinct antiproliferative activity against AGZY83-a and SMMC-7721. A study isolated two compounds: Odorine and Odorinol. Both inhibited carcinogenesis and later promotion stages of skin cancer. [121]

98. CHINESE SALACIA (Salacia chinensis)

Mangiferin, isolated from Salacia chinensis, showed a significant antimutagenic activity suggesting that some triterpenoids might be powerful antioxidants that protect cells against mutagens. A study yielded two new triterpenoids: $7\alpha,21\alpha$-dihydroxyfriedelane-3-one and $7\alpha,29$-dihydroxyfriedelane-3-one plus a known triterpenoid $21\alpha,30$-dihydroxyfriedelane-3-one. The first showed excellent activity against Hep-G2, LU, KB, and MCF-7. [122]

99. CHINESE SARSAPARILLA (Smilax china) *IM

Top Recommended Edible Fruit: Only in moderation as it can become toxic in chronic excess. A study of the rhizome extract showed antiproliferative action against A2780 cells. [123]

100. CHINESE STRAWBERRY (Myrica rubra)

Top Recommended Edible Fruit: This is another rarely seen fruit that is not related to strawberries or raspberries despite a mild resemblance. Prodelphinidin B-2 3,3'-di-O-gallate isolated from the bark showed antiproliferative activity against A549 cells. A study showed that sesquiterpenes from the leaf essential oil selectively increased Doxorubicin accumulation in cancer cells without raising the concentration in normal cells improving the effectiveness and toxicity of this anticancer drug against CaCo-2 cells. Another study showed the leaf essential oil compounds A-Humulene and Trans-Nerolidol decreased adhesion of HT29 cells to collagen leading to diminished tumor invasion and metastasis.[124]

101. CHINESE WEDELIA (Wedelia chinensis)

A study in vivo showed oral administration of an extract impeded the formation of prostate cancer tumors. Exposure of prostate cancer cells induced apoptosis selectively in androgen receptor (AR)-positive prostate cancer cells attributed to the principle active compounds Wedelolactone, Luteolin and Apigenin. A study of an extract showed inhibition of growth of EAC. Another study of various extracts showed anticancer activity. Another study showed a fraction of the extract was cytotoxic to CNE-1 cells. [125]

102. CHRYSANTHEMUM (Chrysanthemum morifolium)

Limited usage recommended – reduces white blood cells in excess: A study evaluated aqueous leaf extracts of ten different cultivars of C. morifolium. The Yellow Coin cultivar showed the maximum (69.85%) tumor inhibition. Another study reports an optimized extraction process of flavonoids from C. morifolium and showed they had inhibitory effects on MKN45 cells.[126]

103. CILANTRO (Coriandrum sativum) *IM

Top Recommended Culinary Spice: Cilantro is the leaves and Coriander is the powdered seeds of the same plant and both are powerful medicine. A study of the leaf showed antiproliferative activity on a breast cancer cell line.[127]

104. CIRCASSIAN BEAN (Adenanthera pavonina)

Top Recommended Edible Plant: Leaves and beans are edible. One study showed anti-tumor effect on DAL in vivo.[417]

105. CLIMBING FIG (Ficus pumila)

A study isolated two compounds: Bergapten and Oxypeucedanin hydrate. Both reduced the occurrence of mutated erythrocytes induced by Mitocin C (a known carcinogen.)[128]

106. CLOVES (Syzygium cumini)

Top Recommended Culinary Spice: Cloves have one of the highest ORAC Scores (antioxidant potency) of any edible plant readily available at most well stocked grocery stores of 290,283. Compared to raw carrots with a score of about 700, the spice is gram for gram roughly 416 TIMES more potent in antioxidant power. The dried flowers of this tree also contain many powerful phytonutrients with a long list of health benefits. One study showed inhibition of growth and cell death in HeLa and SiHa cell lines. Another study showed similar effects against MCF-7 cells. Another study showed a chemoprotective effect against chemically induced skin carcinogenesis. Another study demonstrated very effective protection on mice exposed to Gamma radiation. Pretreatment protected them against radiation sickness and increased survival rate from all exposure intensities tested. [129]

107. CLUB MOSS (Lycopodium clavatum)

An extract showed a significant reduction of tumor incidence in the liver after exposure to a known chemical carcinogen. Another study showed that crude extract is a mixture of about 200 alkaloids and that Lycopodine inhibited growth of HeLa. Another study showed preparations induced apoptosis in cancer cells.[130]

108. COCKSPUR (Pisonia aculeata)

Two independent studies of leaf extracts showed the anti-tumor activity against EAC in vivo. [131]

109. COCONUT (Cocos nucifera) *IM

Top Recommended Edible Seed: The Coconut is actually a fruit with a unique adaptation in that the "fruit pulp" consists of woody fibers and it can float allowing the trees to spread across great distances of open ocean and this is why they are often found along island seashores where the fruits have landed and the seeds have taken root. The seed meat and milk are incredibly nutritious and loaded with powerful RARE Nutritional Fatty Acids: Capric, Caprylic and Lauric Acids that have proven health benefits. One study of aqueous extracts of the husk showed anti-tumor activity against a leukemia cell line. Another study of aqueous extracts showed anti-tumor activity against K562. The cytokinins are considered the most important component of coconut water and have shown anti-aging, anticarcinogenic and antithrombotic effects in numerous studies. The cytokinins identified are N6-Isopentenyladenine, Dihydrozeatin, Trans-Zeatin, Kinetin, Ortho-Topolin, Dihydrozeatin O-Glucoside, Trans-Zeatin O-Glucoside, Trans-Zeatin Riboside, Kinetin Riboside, and Trans-Zeatin Riboside-5'-Monophosphate. Coconut husk is rich in catechins, antioxidant Polyphenols, and a study showed they inhibited proliferation of K562 cells.[37]

110. COLEUS (Plectranthus barbatus) *IM

Top Recommended Holistic Plant: Coleus, a.k.a. C. Forskohlii, is a very popular landscaping plant for its colorful leaves and it is a member of the mint family and related to Basil and Oregano. The active ingredient is in its highest concentrations in the roots, but home preparation is not recommended. Instead find a supplement offering 50 mg per capsule of Forskolin (the active phytonutrient.) Since 1974 scientific studies have shown that Forskolin is a potent immunostimulant, very useful for those undergoing chemotherapy, and it is also very powerful at lowering blood pressure, so much so that if you are on blood pressure medication you must not use Coleus. Coleus also increases stomach acid, so watch for this side effect as well and be prepared to take Milk of Magnesia (#1 antacid because it provides some much needed Magnesium.)[132]

111. COMMON COCKSCOMB (Celosia argentea) *IM
An aqueous extract showed an anti-metastatic effect based on immunomodulatory properties. Another study evaluated the effect of leaves on antioxidant status, PSA, and other hematological indicators in vivo and showed significant decrease in PSA levels and may help inhibit BPH. Another study isolated: Luteolin-7-O-glucoside and 1-(4-hydroxy-2-methoxybenzofuran-5-yl)-3-phenylpropane-1,3-dione. Both exhibited significant antioxidant and cytotoxic activity against SiHa, HCT, and MCF-7. [133]

112. COMMON LEUCAS (Leucas aspera) *IM
A study showed significant anti-tumor activity on DAL in vivo.[134]

113. CONFEDERATE ROSE (Hibiscus mutabilis)
Recommended Holistic Herb: All species of Hibiscus have holistic properties but do not overindulge, they are very powerful medicine and can quickly become toxic with chronic overuse. A study isolated a hexameric 150-kDa lectin from the dried seeds and it showed antiproliferative activity toward HepG2 and MCF-7.[135]

114. COPTIS (Coptis spp.) *IM
Top Recommended Holistic Herb: North American species are endangered, but C. chinensis or Chinese Goldenthread is an adequate substitute. The plants contain Berberine and Coptisine. Berberine has numerous studies showing it to have potent anti-inflammatory and anti-tumor properties.[136]

115. CORAL TREE (Macaranga grandifolia)
Recommended Holistic Herb: This is another holistic plant that may be somewhat difficult to find and be aware that many other plants share the same common name. This plant has many unique phytonutrients and one study isolated a new stilbenoid, Mappain, from a closely related species which proved to be potent and effective against SK-OV-3 and the drug-resistant SKVLB-1 cell line. Another study of the Schweinfurthins (Mappain is similar to Schweinfurthin C, discovered in M. schweinfurthii) showed they are a promising group of anti-tumor compounds.[137]

116. CORDYLINE (Cordyline fruticosa)
Recommended Edible Plant: Cordyline is not just a popular ornamental with its vertical stems tipped in bright red leaves, it is also edible. Young leaf shoots are cooked like a vegetable and in Fiji it is used as a sweetener. The deep red color in the leaves is caused by anthocyanidins, the same class of powerful antioxidants found in cranberries and blueberries and they are what make the leaves powerful medicine. One study isolated Thymidine, which inhibited cell division and reduced cell viability in a human breast

cancer cell line. Another study showed the presence of potential MMK1 inhibitors in the crude extract. [138]

117. CREEPING WOOD SORREL (Oxalis corniculata)
A study of an extract showed significant anti-tumor and antioxidant activities against EAC in vivo.[139]

118. CROWN FLOWER (Calotropis gigantea)
Top Recommended Holistic Herb: At least two studies have confirmed that this plant is non-toxic in high doses and the roots and leaves contain anticancer compounds with superior effect than those regularly used by modern medicine. A study yielded a new compound: Calotropone, together with a known glycoside. The compounds showed inhibitory effects toward K562 and SGC-7901. A study showed the anti-tumor effect of Anhydrosophoradiol-3-acetate (A3A) against EAC in vivo. Another study showed a root extract had antiproliferative activity on HepG2. Another study isolated a new lignan: 9'-Methoxypinoresinol, two new furfurals, and nine known compounds. Compounds 1 and 9 exhibited potent cytotoxicity against PANC-1. Compound 1 also showed significant inhibition of colony formation of PANC-1. Another study isolated two stereoisomeric compounds: Uscharin and a new compound: 1'-epi-uscharin and both showed strong inhibition of HIF-1. [140]

119. CROWN OF THORNS (Euphorbia milii)
Recommended Holistic Herb: This very popular landscape and garden plant is known for its naked heavily thorned vertical gray stems and small red flowers which possess potent antioxidants that have been shown to have anticancer potential against MCF-7 and CaCo-2 cell lines in vivo. [141]

120. CUCUMBER (Cucumis sativus)
Top Recommended Edible Fruit: Most folks don't consider Cucumbers to be fruits, but they are. The Cucumber is the poster child for a very large family of edible vine-borne melons called the Cucurbits which contain compounds called cucurbitacins which have been shown in many studies to have significant anticancer power. The added bonus is that they are also one of the lowest calorie foods as well at just 3.3 cal/oz.[456]

121. CURRY LEAF (Murraya koenigii)
Top Recommended Culinary Spice: As the name suggests, leaves of the tree are used to flavor curry dishes. One study showed anticancer activity against both MCF-7 and MDA-MB-231. A study isolated Girinimbine which showed antiproliferative and apoptotic effects on A549 cells. Another study showed an extract prevented cyclophosphamide-induced DNA damage in bone marrow cells in vivo. Another study of extracts in vivo indicated a protective effect against DAL. Another study in vivo showed Curry Leaf could help prevent human stomach and skin cancers.[142]

122. CUSTARD APPLE (Annona squamosa)
Top Recommended Edible Fruit: A. squamosa and indeed all of the 160+ edible Annona fruits are examples of not judging things

by appearance. All of them are large with big green scales and look like dragon eggs. Inside the pulp is usually white, creamy and delicious. The fruit and the herbal teas made from the leaves of almost every species have great health benefits and are highly recommended although fresh fruit are difficult to find even in South Florida where most of them are grown in the U.S. Fruit extracts showed cytotoxicity against DAL and HeLa cells. The Acetogenins Squadiolin A and B showed potency against HepG2, Hep3B and MCF-7. Six new acetogenins: Annosquacin A to D, Annosquatin A and B were isolated from the seeds and showed potent cytotoxic activity in vitro against five human tumor cell lines. Annosquatin A and B showed high selectivity toward MCF-7 and A549 cell lines. Another study showed seed extracts induced apoptosis in MCF-7 and K562 cells.[143]

123. CUT NUT (Barringtonia acutangula)
A study of extracts showed potent antioxidant and pro-apoptotic activity against the Colo320 cell line.[144]

124. CYNOMETRA (Cynometra ramiflora)
A study of an extract showed selective cytotoxicity against human gastric, colon and breast cancer cell lines. Another study of bark and leaf extracts showed selective cytotoxicity on WiDr. [145]

125. DAINTY SPURS (Rhinacanthus nasutus)
A study isolated three main compounds in the roots: Rhinacanthin C, N, and Q that induced apoptosis of HeLa cells. A study showed anti-tumor cytotoxicity and antiosteoclastogenic activity. This study evaluated Rhinacanthin C, G, N, and Q, and Rhicanthone isolated from the roots. Rhinacanthin C showed the highest anti-tumor activity, with non-apoptotic cell death, and the strongest inhibition of osteoclastogenesis. Another study showed that the root extract had the highest anti-tumor cytotoxicity. [146]

126. DANDELION (Taraxacum officinale)
Top Recommended Holistic Herb: One South Korean study showed decreased cell viability in liver cancer. A study of aqueous extracts from leaves, flowers and roots showed anticarcinogenic activity on breast and prostate cells. Another study showed cytotoxicity and changes in production of cytokines in a human hepatoma cell line. A study showed the root extract specifically and effectively induces apoptosis in human melanoma cells without affecting normal cells. Taraxasterol, a triterpenoid found in high amounts in Dandelion roots, has anti-inflammatory properties and known chemoprotective properties. Chlorogenic and Chicoric Acid are phenolic components of Dandelion in high concentrations and are far more effective antioxidants than the synthetic standard Trolox. [147]

127. DESERT HORSE PURSLANE (Trianthema portulacastrum)
A study showed inhibition of hepatocarcinogenesis in vivo. Another study showed a significant chemoprotective effect against breast cancer. [148]

128. DEVIL'S CLAW (Harpagophytum procumbens)
Top Recommended Holistic Herb: This plant contains Iridoids that are anti-inflammatory; Chlorogenic Acid, Harpagide, Luteolin, Oleanolic Acid, Kaempferol, and the two main active ingredients: Harpagoside and beta-Sitosterol. This is a list of compounds with numerous studies showing them to be effective anticancer agents. USE WITH CAUTION; it earned its name.[149]

129. DEVIL'S TAIL (Polygonum perfoliatum)
A study showed the flavonoids have strong antioxidant activity and one showed moderate anti-tumor activity against PC3 and another inhibited SMMC7721. Another study yielded 8-Oxopinoresinol, which has cytotoxicity against Bcap-37, RKO, SMMC-7721, PC3 and K562 cells.[150]

130. DEVIL'S TONGUE (Sansevieria roxburghiana)
This popular ornamental is easily recognized for its rosette of large sword-like leaves with striking horizontal yellow patchy stripes. A study in vivo showed significant anticancer activity against EAC. Another study of the rhizome extract showed strong anti-tumor activity on EAC mainly due to its antioxidants.[151]

131. DRAGON FRUIT (Hylocereus undatus)
Top Recommended Edible Fruit: It doesn't get much stranger than this one: a cactus with a bizarre-looking edible fruit that tastes wonderful and it is a VINE. It actually needs something to grow up and crawl on and creates a tangle of fleshy four-sided segments covered in thorns. Flowers are sometimes cooked like a vegetable but that would be a severe waste of the excellent fruits that follow them and by the way, like most cacti they need bats to pollinate them. One study showed the antiproliferative activity of an extract on HeLa. Another study showed growth Inhibition and apoptosis on MCF-7 and MDA-MB-435.[153]

132. DRAGON SCALES (Pyrrosia piloselloides)
A study of an extract showed inhibition of cell growth against P388 cells. A study showed cytotoxicity extracts against MCF-7.[154]

133. DRAGON TAIL PLANT (Epipremnum pinnatum)
Two independent studies of the extracts showed growth inhibition against T47D cells. [155]

134. DRUMSTICK TREE (Moringa oleifera)
Top Recommended Edible Plant: The leaves are edible and contain a very high concentration of nutrients: 7 TIMES the Vitamin C of oranges, 4 TIMES the Calcium of milk, 4 TIMES the Vitamin A of carrots, and 3 TIMES the Potassium of bananas. One study showed a seed extract inhibited the formation of EBV-EA induced by TPA (a known carcinogen.) At 100 mcg/ml dosage, the extract inhibited EBV-EA formation by 100% indicating incredible anti-tumor power. Another study showed the chemoprotective effect versus Azoxymethane and Dextran Sodium Sulfate, two well known carcinogens, reducing colon carcinogenesis in vivo. A study showed enhanced cytotoxicity of Cisplatin, a standard anticancer

treatment, and inhibited the growth of PANC-1 cells. Another study of leaf extracts showed significant proliferation reduction of HepG2 and A549 cells. A study showed anticancer potential against MDA-MB-231 and HCT-8. Analysis yielded many known anticancer compounds: Eugenol, Hexadeconoic Acid Ethyl Ester, Isopropyl Isothiocyanate and D-Allose. Another study showed a significant drop in cell proliferation in lung cancer cell lines. [156]

135. DUCK'S EYE (Ardisia elliptica)
Recommended Edible Plant: Leaves, flowers and fruits of this small tree are all edible and it has at least one study showing it to have anticancer properties against the SKBR3 cell line.[157]

136. EAST INDIAN GLOBE THISTLE (Sphaeranthus africanus)
Recommended Holistic/Edible Plant: Leaves of Globe thistle are edible and the plant has powerful health benefits. One study of an extract of the whole plant showed cytotoxicity against various carcinoma cell lines. The isolated flavonoids: Chrysophenol D; 3,7-dimethoxy-4',5,6-trihydroxy flavone; Chrysophenol C; and 3-alpha,5beta-diangeloxoyloxy-7-hydroxycarvotanacetone showed strong antioxidant power.[158]

137. EEL SEAGRASS (Enhalus acoroides)
A study showed the leaf extracts killed 50% of HeLa cells.[159]

138. EGGPLANT (Solanum melongena)
Top Recommended Edible Fruit: This well known fruit is not nearly as popular as it should be. It is very low calorie and loaded with unique beneficial phytochemicals. One study found three steroidal alkaloids: Solasodine, Solamargine and Solasonine plus two steroidal glycosides: β-sitosterol-3-O-β-D-glucoside and Poriferasterol-3-O-β-D-glucoside. The study showed moderate to potent activity against all tested cancer cell lines.[35]

139. EGYPTIAN GRASS (Dactyloctenium aegyptium)
A study of the extracts showed selective growth inhibition against human lung cancer and HeLa cell lines via apoptosis.[160]

140. ELDERBERRY (Sambuca spp.)
Top Recommended Edible Fruit/Holistic Herb: Flowers and leaves contain: Palmitic, Linoleic, and Linolenic Acids, Flavonoids including Rutin, Pectin, and glycosides. Palmitic Acid and Rutin have numerous studies showing their anticancer effectiveness. A Chinese preparation is used for certain forms of pancreatic and liver cancers. The berries and juice are also very good for you and are loaded with antioxidant power which has also been shown in numerous studies to have potent anticancer action.[161]

141. ELEPHANT'S FOOT (Elephantopus mollis)
Both species of Elephantopus in this list are similar in appearance and have the same common name. A study showed E. mollis extract reduced melanogenesis. Another study of an extract showed potent growth inhibition of HepG2 cells. Another study showed it was effective against DLD-1, A549 cells and induced apoptosis in MCF-7 cells. A study yielded three new compounds:

33

Molephantin, Molephantinine, and Phantomolin, and showed they are potent against EAC, Walker-256, and P-388 cell lines.[162]

142. ELEPHANT'S FOOT (Elephantopus scaber)

This odd little weed with clusters of flower buds that look like saucers covered in green spikes that bloom a few at a time has attracted plenty of interest due to its potent anticancer powers. One study isolated four sesquiterpenoids: Deoxyelephantopin, Scabertopin, Isoscabertopin, and Isodeoxyelephantopin. Three showed significant anti-tumor effect in vitro. Another study showed tumor inhibitory activity on skin papillomas in vivo. Another study showed anticancer power on human breast cancer cells. A study isolated Lupeol from the leaves; it reduced viability of MCF-7 cells. Another study of Deoxyelephantopin showed it induced apoptosis and cell cycle arrest in HCT116 cells. A study showed cytotoxicity against HeLa cell lines. A study showed Isodeoxyelephantopin has effective anticancer activity on T47D and A549 cells. Another study showed the cytotoxicity of Isodeoxyelephantopin on human KB. A study showed apoptosis on human epithelial cancer.[454]

143. ENDIVE (Cichorium endivia)

Top Recommended Holistic/Edible Plant: Leaves are edible raw or cooked and have a lot of nutritional and medicinal power. The root extract showed anticancer activity on MCF7 comparable to the standard anticancer drug 5-FU. [163]

144. ENOKI MUSHROOM (Flammulina veluptis) *IM

Top Recommended Edible Mushroom: All edible mushrooms bring beta-Glucans, shown in numerous studies to be powerful immunostimulants and anticancer agents. Most of the gourmet mushrooms have much higher concentrations of the beta-Glucans than Button Mushrooms (in this list) and each species also brings its own unique forms of beta-Glucans which can have dramatic differences in both potency and specific health benefits and they all come highly recommended including store bought Button or Portabella mushrooms. [22][30][74][106][332]

145. EUCALYPTUS (Eucalyptus globulus)

Top Recommended Holistic Herb: Eucalyptus, Aloe and Ginger are the Big 3 of Holistic herbs and are likely the most well known medicinal plants on Earth and for good reason. There are over 300 species of Eucalyptus and they all share similar phytochemistry and substitutions are acceptable. E. globulus "Blue Gum Tree" is the most potent of them all. One study of the leaves of E. robusta identified a new sesquiterpenoid derivative, Euglobal-IIIa, which showed cytotoxicity against five human cancer cell lines.[164]

146. FALSE DAISY (Eclipta prostata)

Top Recommended Edible Plant: Young shoots and leaves are cooked like a vegetable. Testing shows no measurable toxicity and it is loaded with antioxidants and cancer fighting phytochemicals. A study showed antiproliferative and antimetastatic properties on HepG2 and A498 cell lines. A study showed arrested growth and apoptosis in lung cancer cells. Another study showed an extract was selectively cytotoxic to breast cancer cells over noncancerous breast epithelial cells. A study showed anticancer activity on most cell lines tested but showed significant apoptosis on human breast cancer cells. It also inhibited migration of MCF-7 and MDA-MB-231 cells. [165]

147. FALSE GARLIC (Pachyptera alliacea)
A study of the extract of the flowers showed growth inhibition on estrogen receptor positive and estrogen receptor negative breast cancer cells.[166]

148. FALSE HEATHER (Cuphea hyssopifolia)
A study isolated Cuphilin D1 (CD1), a new tannin, which showed antitumor activity in vivo and in vitro. Further study showed cytotoxicity against HL-60. A study isolated four tannins: Cuphiin D1, Cuphiin D2, Cenothein B and Woodfordin C; all significantly inhibited growth of KB, HeLa, DU-145, Hep3B and HL-60. [167]

149. FALSE PRIMROSE (Ludwigia octovalvis) *IM
A study yielded three new triterpenes, which all showed significant cytotoxicity against KB and HT-29.[168]

150. FENNEL (Foeniculum vulgare)
Top Recommended Culinary Spice/Edible Plant: Ground Fennel seed is another widely available spice with enormous health benefit potential. The whole plant, rhizome, stems and leaves are also edible and have a long history of herbal medicinal usage. One study showed selective anti-tumor activity of an extract against B16F10 cells and is cytoprotective to normal cells. Another study showed apoptotic activity against HeLa.[169]

151. FEVER BARK (Alstonia scholaris) *IM
A. scholaris is very popular in holistic medicine but overindulgence is not recommended as it can become toxic in excess. A study of bark extract showed pretreatment provides protection against DNA damage in bone marrow cells caused by radiation. Another study showed it was effective in the early stages of EAC. Another study showed that it inhibited mutagenicity induced by Benzo-a-pyrene in vivo. An anticancer study of an alkaloid fraction in vivo showed an increase in antineoplastic activity and a decline in viable cells versus: HeLa, HepG2, HL60, KB, MCF-7 and EAC. Another study showed effective prevention of DBMA-induced skin tumors in vivo. Another study showed pretreatment enhanced the effectiveness of radiotherapy making HeLa and KB in particular, more vulnerable while protecting healthy cells resulting in DISEASE FREE mice at the end of the study. A study evaluated eight triterpenoids and five sterols. Ursolic acid, Betulinic Acid, Betulin, and $2\beta,3\beta,28$-lup-20 (29)-ene-triol showed antiproliferative activity on A549. Another study showed a bark extract could be effective treatment against leukemia and lymphoma and potential for use as an antioxidant in dietary supplements. Another study showed effective prevention of Bleomycin-induced DNA damage and noted that some compounds

in the bark may enhance DNA repair. Another study demonstrated anticarcinogenic and antimutagenic activity on Methyl Methane Sulfonate-induced damage of bone marrow cells and peripheral human lymphocyte cultures. [170]

152. FINGER GRASS (Limnophila aromatica)

Recommended Edible Plant: An unusual cousin to many other edible grasses, this one has serrated red leaves, smells of turpentine and tastes like lemon. It is eaten raw or cooked in its native range. One study showed cytotoxicity effects on Jurkat, MCF7, and HepG2.[171]

153. FISH FERN (Blechnum orientale)

Top Recommended Edible Plant: It was only a matter of time before I found a plant that produces EPA – Eicosapentaenoic Acid, one of the Omega-3 Fatty acids normally only found in fish. So here it is: a plant that can provide some EPA which is outstanding news for the Vegans and young tender fronds are eaten like a vegetable too. Just get professional verification that you have the correct species. One study showed the roots have high cytotoxicity against MCF-7. Another study showed a leaf extract had cytotoxic activity on HT-29. Another study isolated a proanthocyanidin which showed selective cytotoxicity against HT-29 cells. In another study of five medicinal ferns, B. orientale had the highest concentration of proanthocyanidin and showed cytotoxicity toward K562.[172]

154. FIREFLY MANGROVE (Sonneratia caseolaris)

A study isolated 24 compounds. An in-vitro cytotoxic assay against SMMC-7721 showed 3',4',5,7-tetrahydroxyflavone had significant anticancer activity.[173]

155. FIVE-LEAF CHASTE TREE (Vitex negundo)

Extracts of the leaves showed anti-tumor effect against DAL. [174]

156. FLAME VINE (Pyrostegia venusta)

A study showed the anti-tumor activity of flower extracts against B16F10-Nex2 cells in vivo. The main components, Octasane and Triacontane, appeared promising anti-tumor compounds.[175]

157. FLAMINGO BILL (Sesbania grandiflora)

Recommended Edible Plant: Named for the pendulous flowers that resemble Flamingo bills before they open which are edible raw or steamed as are the cooked long string bean pods that follow. One study showed tumor growth inhibition against EAC comparable to the standard drug 5-FU. Another study isolated a novel protein from the flower which inhibited cell proliferation and induced apoptosis in DAL and SW-480. Another study showed the anticancer power of the leaves via apoptosis especially against A549. Another study showed apoptotic and autophagic effects of the flowers against a human leukemia cell line. [176]

158. FLAX SEED (Linum usitatissimum)

Top Recommended Edible Seed: Flaxseed is a rich source of ALA – Alpha-Linoleic Acid, the plant Omega-3. It is also high in Omega-6 fatty acids which have also been shown to have potent health benefits. Flaxseed has been shown to slow breast cancer by blocking estrogen receptors in the cancer cells due to the plant's high levels of phytoestrogens. [14][17][38]

159. FOUR O'CLOCK (Mirabilis jalapa)

A study of leaf fractions with RIP properties showed cytotoxic activity against a breast cancer cell line. Another study isolated a 30 kDA protein fraction with RIP properties which caused selective cytotoxic effect on breast and cervical cancer cells. Another study showed potent anticancer activity of proteins of the plant.[178]

160. FRAGRANT GLORY BOWER (Clerodendrum chinense)

All species of Clerodendrum are large bushes with showy displays of clusters of beautiful flowers and this species is very popular for its tight clusters of pale pink rose-like flowers. One study showed that C. chinense may also be the source of an effective treatment for acute myelocytic leukemia.[179]

161. FRAGRANT PREMNA (Premna odorata)

A study showed an extract to be a significant hepatoprotective by decreasing serum enzymes, Bilirubin and lipid peroxidation, as well as Silymarin. It also showed significant anti-tumor cytotoxicity. Another study showed it to be highly cytotoxic against HCT116, MCF-7 and A549 cell lines.[180]

162. FRANGIPANI (Plumeria acuminata)

TOXIC: Six constituents were isolated from Frangipani bark which showed cytotoxic activity against breast, colon, fibrosarcoma, lung, melanoma, and KB. Another study of the leaf extract yielded: Stigmast-7-enol, Lupeol Carboxylic Acid, and Ursolic Acid. The first reduced the mutagenic effect of Mitomycin C. Another study showed the anti-tumor and antioxidant properties of leaf extract on EAC in vivo.[181]

163. FRANKINCENSE (Boswellia thurifera)

Top Recommended Holistic Herb: A legendary healing herb since ancient times, Frankincense is generally used as a topical analgesic. It contains: Bassorin, Boswellic Acid, and Alibanoresin and it has been shown to be a very powerful anti-inflammatory that uses unique pathways which may also be effective against certain forms of cancer as well.[182]

164. FROGFRUIT (Phyla nodiflora)

Recommended Holistic Herb: The fruit is weird, like a small acorn shaped purple honeycomb, but the plant is loaded with powerful phytonutrients. One study showed the anti-tumor activity of an extract on EAC in vivo. Another study showed anticancer power against MCF7. Another study of extracts showed inhibition of MCF-7 cell growth. A study showed the anticancer effect of leaf extracts on NCI-H460 cells. Another study of the extracts showed profound inhibition and DNA fragmentation in MCF-7 cells.[183]

165. GALANGAL (Kaempferia galanga)

Recommended Medicinal Herb: This lily has a long sordid history as a dangerous narcotic, but it is not as bad as its reputation. On the contrary, Galangal is a truly orchid-like lily with broad dark green leaves and it has a very well known and powerful anticancer agent in the rhizomes called P-methoxycinnamate which is getting a lot of attention in medical science. The plant has also passed at least one test showing that it is not toxic even in much exaggerated doses. One study of plant rhizomes used in traditional Malaysian medicine showed it inhibits chemically induced carcinomas. Both cis- and trans- ethyl-p-methoxycinnamate, isolated from Galangal, have strong anticarcinogenic effect. Another study showed an oil fraction from the extract increased apoptosis in colon cancer in vivo. [184]

166. GALANGAL GINGER (Alpinia galanga) *IM
Recommended Culinary Herb: This oddball has a lot of chemistry similar to true Galangal (Kaempferia galanga) but it is a distinct species actually more closely related to ginger. One study showed inhibition and cytotoxicity to PC3. Another study showed inhibition of breast adenocarcinoma cells. [185]

167. GARDENIA (Gardenia jasminoides)
Top Recommended Edible Plant: Gardenia flowers are added to herbal teas for the fragrance but they contain potent and unique phytonutrients that have shown many health benefits. However, moderation is advised. A study showed Genipin induces apoptosis and inhibits invasive and migratory abilities of the highly invasive MDA-MB-231 cell line. Another study showed strong anticancer effect against HepG2 cells.[186]

168. GARLIC (Allium sativum)
Top Recommended Culinary Spice: Better cooked than raw and loaded with Chromium that is difficult to get in 100% RDA amounts on a daily basis, add the minced cloves of this "sulfur lily" to soups, stews, casseroles, and even Oil and Vinegar dressing. Studies have shown that glucosinolates are powerful medicine and help with blood pressure, blood sugar and cholesterol levels, proper maintenance of cartilage and joints, and even help fight some forms of cancer. In a clinical study on stomach and colorectal cancer prevention using 3.5 grams to 30 grams of fresh or cooked garlic per week determined that the effect in stomach cancers was probably through its inhibitory effect on H. pylori (bacteria that can survive in the stomach and cause ulcers and cancer.) Another review of many studies noted that Garlic does play a role in cancer prevention likely due to the presence of high concentrations of sulfur compounds. Another study showed Garlic may support defense mechanisms against induced carcinogenesis in salivary glands in vivo by increasing the availability and/or utilization of beta-Carotene. Another study showed diallyl sulfide, another glucosinolate found in garlic, reduced the incidence rate of chemically induced colorectal adenocarcinoma. Another study of Black garlic (processed from ordinary white garlic in temperature and humidity controlled conditions) showed enhanced anti-tumor

potency. Aged black garlic yielded an increased amount of amino acids and S-allyl-L-cysteine which might have contributed to the anti-tumor potency. Aged and odorless garlic products are missing Allicin which is believed to have significant health benefits. [10]

169. GERBERA DAISY (Gerbera jamesonii)

Recommended Holistic Herb: An in vitro study showed selective antiproliferative and antimetastatic activity on A549 cells.[187]

170. GHOST FLOWER (Aeginetia indica) *IM

Top Recommended Holistic Herb: This is one of the few holistic herbs that has shown a very rare property: the ability to make mice IMMUNE to exposure to a tumorous cell line. Once administered, the treatment, they were CURED of the cancer they already had and when REEXPOSED to it, (without any further treatments of the herb) they did not get the cancer again. I am not saying that this herb cures cancer, or that it can make humans immune to the type of cancer in the TWO studies that made these findings, but it is one of the most exciting plants in terms of what looks like it can do and experimentally CONFIRMED conclusions in this entire list. One study isolated a 55kDa protein from the seed extract and strongly suggested that it is a potent Th1 inducer and may be a strong immunotherapeutic for patients with malignant diseases. Another study investigated the effect of this Traditional Chinese Medicinal herb, on renal cancer and found a synergistic effect on cytotoxicity when combined with 5-FU possibly through alteration of chemical resistance related genes. Another study of the seed extract in vivo against Meth A tumor cells found it promoted development of antigen-specific IMMUNITY IN THE CURED mice. Another study isolated the 55kDa protein, AILb-A, from the seed extract and showed it induces a Th1-type T-cell response causing a marked anti-tumor effect. The results suggest pathways of TUMOR IMMUNITY that are induced by the plant-derived protein AILb-A.[188]

171. GIN BERRY (Glycosmis pentaphylla)

Recommended Edible Fruit: But the medicinal qualities come from extracts of the leaves, stems, roots and bark of the plant. A study isolated four sulfur-containing amides: E-dambullin, Z-dambullin, E-methyldambullin and Z-methyldambulin which were strongly cytotoxic against a T-lymphoblastic leukemia cell line. A study showed anticancer and apoptosis against Hep3B.[189]

172. GINGER (Zingiber officinale) *IM

Top Recommended Culinary Spice: Ginger is one of the BIG 3 holistic herbs of notoriety with Aloe and Eucalyptus. The claimed properties of Ginger are impressive, and possibly exaggerated, but no one doubts that it is powerful medicine. A study showed Ginger may exert its anticancer effect by replacing the action of normal oxidant/antioxidant pathways within cells. The extract significantly reduced the expression of proinflammatory markers in liver cancer in vivo. Another study showed that many diarylheptanoids and gingerol-related compounds in the rhizome possess significant antiproliferative activity on HL-60. Another study showed ginger extract and 6-Gingerol both directly interfere with colon cancer proliferation. A study of an extract against Cholangiocarcinoma in vivo showed promising anticancer activity and no toxicity. A study showed terpenoids in the distilled extract of ginger are potent antiproliferative agents against endometrial cancer cells. [190]

173. GLABROUS SARCANDRA (Sarcandra glabra)
A study showed S. glabra prevented thrombocytopenia; a possible complication caused by the anticancer drug 5-FU. Another study showed selective growth inhibition on various cancer cell lines with the best results on HL-60. Another study showed extracts have an anti-tumor effect against nasopharyngeal carcinoma in vivo.[191]

174. GLOBE AMARANTHUS (Gomphrena globosa)
Top Recommended Holistic Herb: The flowers are added to herbal teas or used alone. They contain betacyanins that are also found in Beets which are powerful antioxidants and have shown a wide range of health benefits. One study showed the anticancer activity of an extract against EAC. A study showed anticancer properties against DAL and EAC cell lines. The active compound possessing the anticancer activity against human cancer cell lines MCF-7, DU 145, HeLa and A-431 was found to be Oleuropein also found in olives. [192]

175. GOAT WEED (Ageratum conyzoides)
A study of extracts against NSCLC, colon adenocarcinoma, gastric carcinoma and breast carcinoma showed the plant has anticancer properties.[193]

176. GOJI BERRY (Lycium chinense)
Top Recommended Edible Fruit: Most "Goji berries" that you will find are actually Wolfberries (L. barbatum) which is very similar, but not the real thing. Wolfberries are much more popular with suppliers because the bushes are larger and produce a lot more berries than the true Goji Berry bush. Studies have shown that Goji Berries can improve immune function and help fight certain forms of cancer including skin cancer.[457]

177. GOLD DUST DRACAENA (Dracaena surculosa)
A study isolated three new saponins: Surculoside A, B and C, and evaluated them against HL-60 cells.[194]

178. GOLDEN EYE GRASS (Curculigo orchioides) *IM
Top Recommended Edible Plant: Aside from being edible fresh, supplements are also available and the plant has several unique and powerful phytochemicals that give it potent anticancer powers. Chronic high dosages are not recommended. A study showed tumor reduction against DAL. A study showed the anti-tumor effect of polysaccharides from the plant on HeLa cells.[195]

179. GOLDEN LEATHER FERN (Acrostichum aureum)
In a study of 16 plants against human gastric, colon, and breast cancer, A. aureum showed the strongest selective cytotoxicity.

Another study showed strong selective cytotoxicity against cancer cells. The study isolated: Di-(2-Methylheptyl)phthalate and (2S,3S)-Sulfated Pterosin C which showed very potent cytotoxicity against all tested cell lines. A study isolated three compounds identified as new natural products. Eight known compounds were isolated for the first time: Di-(2-Methylheptyl)Phthalate, (2S, 3S)-Pterosin C, (2R)-Pterosin P, Tetracosane, Quercetin-3-O-B-D-Glucosyl-(6→1)-A-L-Rhamnoside, Quercetin-3-O-A-L-Rhamnosyl-7-O-B-D-Glucoside, Quercetin-3-O-A-L-Rhamnoside, and Patriscabratine. One of the new compounds showed the strongest cytotoxicity on gastric and colon adenocarcinoma cell lines.[196]

180. GOLDEN ROD (Solidago virgaurea)
Despite its powerful phytochemicals and relatively low toxicity, excessive usage of Goldenrod is DANGEROUS to the kidneys; CAUTION IS ADVISED. Ironically its primary usage in holistic medicine is to treat Urinary Tract Infections and Kidney stones. One study showed cytotoxicity on a prostate cancer cell line in vivo. Another study showed that an active component of Golden Rod inhibits FAS activity and induces apoptosis in the prostate tumor cells.[197]

181. GOTU KOLA (Centella asiatica)
Top Recommended Holistic Herb/Edible Plant: The leaves are edible raw and the plant is legendary for its health benefits. One study showed immunomodulatory action of extracts and suggested potential as a chemoprotective and anticancer agent. Another study showed an extract was a strong defense against Hydrogen Peroxide induced DNA damage. Another study showed apoptosis in CaCo-2 cell lines.[198]

182. GOVERNOR'S PLUM (Flacourtia indica)
Top Recommended Edible Fruit: Governor's Plum is uncommon, but it is edible. A study showed antiproliferative and pro-apoptotic effects against HCT116 cells.[199]

183. GRAPES (Vitis vinifera)
Top Recommended Edible Fruit: Grapes, particularly dark ones like Concord, are loaded with anthocyanidins which are powerful antioxidants with a host of health benefits. Grapes also contain Resveratrol which has been shown to inhibit three molecular processes in cells that could lead to anti-aging potency. Myricetin, also found in grapes, is both a powerful antioxidant and a pro-oxidant at the same time that helps fight viruses; and the list goes on. Many of these compounds have studies showing that they have anticancer activity as well.[9]

184. GREATER PLANTAIN (Plantago major)
Top Recommended Edible Plant: Not to be confused with the large starchy banana, this is a small leafy herb and all parts are edible. Leaves are eaten raw in salad or cooked like a vegetable. Few such plants (little green leafy weeds) are actually nutritious but this one is loaded with Thiamine and Riboflavin and it has

anticancer power. Two independent studies demonstrated efficacy against EAC. Another study showed broad spectrum activities against leukemia, carcinomas and viruses, as well as assisting immune response. Another study showed protection against Azoxymethane-induced ACF cancer.[200]

185. GREEN PEA (Pisum sativum)

Top Recommended Edible Plant: Common green peas are nutritious, low calorie, high fiber, bring plenty of molybdenum and essential amino acids and might help fight cancer too. One study showed activity against CaSki cell lines. Another study in Mexico showed that 2mg Coumestrol per day can significantly reduce the risk of at least one form of stomach cancer (1 cup of Green Peas contains about 10mg of Coumestrol.)[16]

186. GUAVA (Psidium guajava) *IM

Top Recommended Edible Fruit: Guavas have a higher concentration of Vitamin C per ounce, per calorie and per cost than any citrus fruit and they bring unique phytonutrients with health benefits as well. One study showed extracts to be effective in preventing tumor development. Another study showed that Guava was 4 TIMES more potent than the approved anticancer drug Vincristine against KB cells. Another study showed the antiproliferative effect of guava fruit extract against various cancer cell lines. Another study in vivo used a combination of bark, leaf, and root extract to inhibit growth of B16 cells. A study of dried Guava extract found high levels of phenolics, flavonoids, and antioxidants suggesting guava has anti-tumor potential.[81]

187. GUAZUMA (Guazuma ulmifolia)

A study showed three plants inhibited HeLa cell growth: Gmelina arborea, Guazuma ulmifolia, and Curculigo orchioides.[201]

188. HEAL-ALL (Prunella vulgaris)

Top Recommended Holistic Herb: Heal-all has a reputation for literally being able to heal all possible afflictions. While that might be a stretch, it contains Betulinic Acid, D-Camphor, Delphinidin, Hyperoside, Oleanolic Acid, Rosmarinic Acid, Rutin, and Ursolic Acid most of which have at least one study each showing that they have anticancer properties.[202]

189. HEARTLEAF HEMPVINE (Mikania cordata)

A study showed that the presence of chemical carcinogens is reduced by enhancement (from compounds in this plant) of drug-detoxifying enzymes in the liver. Another study showed selective cytotoxicity against MCF-7 cells. [203]

190. HENNA (Lawsonia inermis)

One study showed tumor suppression against gluteal sarcoma. Another study Showed that the unique compounds in the leaf have a profound inhibition (>88%) of EBV-EA in the Raji cell line.[415]

191. HEN'S EYES (Ardisia crenata)

A study showed Ardisiacrispin A and B inhibited proliferation of Bel-7402 cells. A study found nine compounds: 5-Hydroxymethyl-

2-Furalclehyde, Ethyl-Beta-D-Fructopyranoside, Syringic Acid, N-Butyl-Beta-D-Fructofuranoside, N-Butyl-Alpha-D-Fructofuranoside, Methyl-Alpha-D-Fructofuran-oside, (+)-Bergenin, Ardisiacrispin B, Asperuloside Acid. All of these showed anti-tumor anti-metastatic activities. [204]

192. HOLLY-LEAVED ACANTHUS (Acanthus ilicifolius)

A study showed a leaf extract prevented hepatic DNA damage in tumor-bearing mice. Another study found an extract to be effective against tumor progression and skin papillomagenesis in vivo. A study showed effective anticancer treatment of EAC in vivo. A study yielded an extract of the flowers with high antioxidant power suggesting potential for cancer therapy. Another study showed highly effective cancer prevention and antioxidant health benefits against hydrocortisone-induced genotoxicity in vivo. [205]

193. HOLY BASIL (Ocimum tenuiflorum) *IM

Top Recommended Holistic Herb: Considered sacred in the Hindu religion, Holy Basil, a close relative to culinary Basil, has a long list of proven health benefits including immunomodulatory effects as well as helping fight various forms of cancer with its powerful array of phytochemicals and antioxidants. Administration of extracts in vivo against sarcoma tumors resulted in a significant reduction in tumor volume and increase in lifespan. A review cites various scientific studies on the anticancer activity of Holy Basil against: lung, skin, oral, cervical, gastric, breast, and prostate cancers. Another study showed inhibitory effect on MDA-MB-435 and MCF-10A. A study showed anticancer activity on MCF-7. A study showed an extract inhibited proliferation, migration, invasion, and induced apoptosis of pancreatic cancer cells in vitro. [206]

194. HORSETAIL (Equisetum arvense)

A study of an extract showed cytotoxic effects on U937 cells. Another study found flavonoids, mainly Isoquercetin, which exhibited significant cytotoxicity on HeLa cancer cells. [207]

195. HOG PLUM (Spondias pinnata)

Top Recommended Edible Fruit: There are many species of Spondias that produce edible fruits that mostly go under the name "Hog Plum." Not as nutritious as many other fruits in this list but they still have antioxidants and potential health benefits. One study of a bark extract showed anticancer potential against A549 and MCF-7. Another study evaluated the major constituent compounds for anticancer power against U87 cells. Methyl gallate was shown to be a potent antioxidant that induces apoptosis in U87. [82]

196. HONEY

Top Recommended Sweetener: This is the ONLY animal based product in this list, but it makes the grade for many reasons. It is superior to processed white cane sugar which has been shown to increase the risk of cancer, and many artificial sweeteners like saccharin are PROVEN CARCINOGENS. Honey has a very high Glycemic index of about 70, but the complex sugars provide fuel to the liver and it brings Pinocembrin, Pinostrobin and Chrysin, three powerful flavonoid antioxidants. Pinocembrin has studies showing that it supports enzyme activity and causes apoptosis in certain cancer cell lines. [458]

197. HONEYBUSH (Cyclopia spp.) *IM
Top Recommended Holistic Herb: A caffeine-free red tea is made from Honeybush and while there are no direct scientific studies of the plant, it does contain polyphenols which have been shown to have anti-tumor activity.[208]

198. HUMMINGBIRD BUSH (Hamelia patens) *IM
Be very careful that you are getting the correct species because MANY different plants are called "Hummingbird bush." In a study of nine plants for cytotoxic activity, the root bark of H. patens had the highest anticancer activity on HeLa cells.[209]

199. INDIAN HELIOTROPE (Heliotropium indicum) *IM
Two studies showed the anti-tumor effects of Indicine N-Oxide on tumors including carcinosarcoma, leukemia, and melanoma. A study showed antiproliferative activity against a human breast adenocarcinoma cell line. Another study showed cytotoxicity on HeLa. Another study showed cytotoxicity of a leaf extract against the NCI-H226 cell line.[407]

200. INDIAN HEMP (Hibiscus cannabinus)
Also called Kenaf, the Seed extract and Seed oil both showed significant anticancer activity against all cell lines tested including human cervical, breast, colon and lung cancer cells. [210]

201. INDIAN MANGROVE (Avicennia officinalis)
A study showed the anticancer activity of leaf extract on EAC.[211]

202. INDIAN MARSHWEED (Limnophila indica)
Two independent studies showed no toxicity on healthy cells but selective cytotoxicity against breast and gastric cancer cells. [212]

203. INDIAN PATCHOULI (Pogostemon heyneanus)
A study showed cytotoxicity on MCF-7 and MDA-MB-231. [213]

204. INDIAN SNOWBERRY (Breynia vitis-idaea)
A study of leaf extracts showed anticancer activity in HEPG2 cell lines. The extracts were found to be nontoxic. [214]

205. INDIAN ZEHNERIA (Zehneria japonica)
This is yet another member of the vine borne melons or Cucurbits. It is edible but it appears to act like a purgative thus it is not very well known or cultivated. At least one study has shown anticancer activity against leukemia and prostate cancer cells.[215]

206. INDIGO (Indigofera tinctoria) *IM
Traditional Chinese Medicine: Used to treat chronic myelocytic leukemia. One study showed a fraction of an extract of the aerial parts of the plant was antiproliferative on A549 cells. Indirubin has been isolated as a minor constituent and studies have shown Indirubin inhibits cyclin-dependent kinases in tumor cells. Another study suggested the inhibition of CDK activity in human tumor cells is a major mechanism by which Indirubin derivatives exert potent

antitumor action. Another study showed Indirubin inhibits MCF-7 cell growth. Another study of leaf extract showed cytotoxicity on NCI-H69. Another study of extracts showed potent anticancer activity on: HCT116, NCI-H460, and U251 cancer cell lines. [216]

207. INSULIN PLANT (Chamaecostus cuspidatus)

A study showed cytotoxicity of crude extracts against HL60, Jurkat and THP-1 cancer cell lines.[217]

208. IRONWEED (Vernonia cinereum)

Top Recommended Holistic Herb: This innocuous little weed is a powerhouse of antioxidants and other beneficial phytonutrients. That should come as no surprise since all weeds are so successful because they have perfected the art of resisting harmful bacteria, fungi, and viruses and grow rapidly and reproduce quickly all of which leads to them being packed with strong phytonutrients. Ironweed has two studies showing anticancer potential. One reduced tumor mass in DAL and the other inhibited metastasis of lung tumors.[218]

209. IRONWOOD TREE (Memecylon ovatum)

A study showed the antiproliferative and pro-apoptotic activity of a leaf extract on gastric cancer cells. Another study showed potent antioxidant activity that neutralized hydroxyl radicals indicating that it can protect DNA.[219]

210. IVORY MAHOGANY (Dysoxylum decandrum)

A crude leaf extract showed high cytotoxicity against MCF-7 and HT-29 cells. Analysis yielded Squalene and beta-Sitosterol, both well known anticancer agents.[220]

211. IVY-RUE (Zanthoxylum rhetsa)

The analysis of the bark isolated two lignans: Yangambin and Kobusin, a berberine alkaloid: Columbamine, and a triterpenoid: Lupeol. Kobusin showed cytotoxicity against B16F10 cells.[221]

212. IXORA (Ixora coccinea) *IM

Top Recommended Holistic Herb: Ixora is popular worldwide as a landscape ornamental with its large clusters of small red flowers. One study of an extract of the flowers showed activity on ascitic tumors. It was selectively cytotoxic with no toxicity toward normal lymphocytes but high toxicity on human leukemic lymphocytes. A study yielded Ixorapeptide 1 and Ixorapeptide 2. The first showed selective potency against Hep3B. Kaempferol and Luteolin from the plant inhibited collagen-induced platelet aggregation. Flowers have shown inhibition of tumor growth and increased life span against DAL and EAC in vivo. Who knew this common shrub could possibly help fight cancer?[222]

213. JABOTICABA (Myrciaria cauliflora)

Top Recommended Edible Fruit: Perhaps you prefer to call it "Brazilian Tree Grape," this unusual, rare, and difficult to grow relative to the common Cherry Hedge plant yields fruits that taste like grapes and have very powerful antioxidants and other phytonutrients. One study showed a seed extract had very high antioxidant activity and antiproliferative effects against human oral carcinoma cell lines. Another study showed protective action of Pedunculagin against chemical-induced micronuclei and DNA damage of bone marrow cells in vivo indicating that the seed extract is both chemoprotective and induces DNA repair.[223]

214. JACKFRUIT (Artocarpus heterophyllus)

Top Recommended Edible Fruit: Artocarpus is a vast genus of over 50 fruiting trees most of which are not just edible but also delicious. The trees are also usually quite large as are their fruits and Jackfruit is the largest tree-borne fruit on Earth weighing in at over 80 lbs and measuring up to 4 feet long and over a foot in diameter. It is often described as a cross between pineapple and banana and is highly prized in its native countries worldwide. One study showed an extract to be cytotoxic on Hep2 cells. Another study of an extract showed excellent cytotoxicity against the A549 cell line, but no activity against HeLa or MCF-7 cell lines. Another study showed Jacalin, a protein from Jackfruit seed, had activity against MCF-7 and H1299. Another study showed crude leaf extracts had significant cytotoxicity against MCF-7 and MDA-MB-231 cell lines.[224]

215. JAMAICAN CHERRY (Muntingia calabura)

Top Recommended Edible Fruit: Well known in Jamaica but rarely seen outside of its native habitat, this fruit is said to be exquisite and it is very healthy too. One study isolated 12 new flavonoids and most were cytotoxic and some exhibited selective activity against a number of human cancer cell lines. Another study showed the leaves possess potential antiproliferative and antioxidant activities attributed to high phenolic content. Another study of a fruit extract yielded constituents with previously known biological activities: Squalene (chemoprotective against colon carcinogenesis); Linoleic Acid (anticancer agent); beta-Sitosterol (antiproliferative against MCF-7 and MDA-MB-231); Stigmasterol (effective against EAC.) Another study showed strong cytotoxicity of leaf extract against HL60.[225]

216. JAPANESE ALNUS (Alnus japonica)

A study showed extracts have antioxidant and anticancer effects on AGS cell lines.[226]

217. JASMINE (Jasminum sambac)

Top Recommended Holistic Herb: There are many species of Jasmine and most share similar phytochemistry and can be substituted for one another. One study of an extract showed significant antiproliferative activity on DAL in vitro and in vivo. Another study showed anticancer activity against DAL comparable to the standard drug 5-FU.[227]

218. JAVA BRUCEA (Brucea javanica)

One study reported anticancer activity of the water extract on four cancer cell lines: A549, Hep3B, MDA-MB-231, and SLMT-1. The researchers noted that the B. javanica extract causes cancer cell death through a mitochondrial dependent pathway associated with Caspase 3 activation.[413]

219. JOB'S TEARS (Coix lacryma-jobi)

Top Recommended Grain: A study of the isolated compounds showed anti-tumor activity attributed to: Palmitic, Stearic, Oleic and Linoleic acids. Another study showed anticancer activity against breast and skin cancer. Another study of extracts showed antiproliferative and inhibitory effects, attributed mainly to Caffeic and Chlorogenic acid, on a gastric cancer cell line. Another study yielded six compounds with very strong antimutagenic activity: p-Hydroxybenzaldehyde, Vanillin, Syringaldehyde, Sinapaldehyde, trans-Coniferylaldehyde, and Coixol. Two had potent antioxidant activity and trans-Coniferylaldehyde may be highly promising for cancer prevention. Another study of the triterpene-loaded seed oil showed effective anti-tumor activity against Lewis lung cancer and was as effective as a standard drug but with lower general toxicity. A study induced apoptosis in MCF-7 attributed to Triolein.[229]

220. JOE-PYE WEED (Eupatorium purpureum)

Top Recommended Holistic Herb: All that remains in history of the Native American medicine man Joe Pye who traveled colonial America healing Typhus fever, is his name on this plant which is said to be the foundation of his remedies. A close relative to Boneset, E. purpureum is believed to have potent anticancer powers likely due to the presence of many flavonoids including Eupatorin.[230]

221. JOSHUA TREE (Yucca spp.) *IM

Top Recommended Holistic Herb: This desert plant's roots have saponins which have been shown in studies and even applied medicine manufacture to have immunostimulant and anti-tumor properties. Yucca is best taken in product capsules with specific dosages because saponins can turn toxic in excess.[231]

222. JUDAS EAR (Auricularia auricula-judae)

Top Recommended Edible Mushroom: The edible mushrooms are all under investigation for their enormous potential health benefits mainly due to their unique polysaccharides called beta-Glucans which have potent anti-cancer, tumor inhibitory and immunostimulant properties. One study compared the anti-tumor activities of two (1→3)-beta-D-glucans isolated from the fruiting body of A. auricula-judae. Another study showed the anti-tumor activity of extracts from A. auricula-judae on P388D1 cells. A fraction from A. auricula-judae showed anti-tumor activity against bronchoalveolar and gastric cancer cells. Another study showed the anti-tumor activities of two different (1→3)-beta-D-glucans and other branched polysaccharides against implanted S-180 solid tumors in vivo. [74][228]

223. JUJUBE (Ziziphus jujuba) *IM

Top Recommended Edible Fruit: The candy was actually named after the fruit which is sundried and gets the consistency of gummy candy is said to taste like dates. One study showed the anticancer activity of Jujube against HepG2. A study of aqueous fruit extract showed preventive effects against anemia and other complications of MDA-MB-468 cell line cancer. Studies show Jujubes are rich in compounds which have antiproliferative and anticancer effects including triterpenoid acids and polysaccharides [232]

224. JUTE (Corchorus capsularis)
While edible, the plant increases blood pressure and should be taken in limited quantities. Galactolipid 1 has been shown to be responsible for the anti-tumor activity of Jute.[233]

225. KALANCHOE (Kalanchoe laciniata)
Three independent studies have shown that extracts of Kalanchoe have antiproliferative effects on MCF-7 and CaCo-2 cells.[418]

226. KAMALA (Mallotus philippensis)
A study showed root extracts were antiproliferative against p53-deficient HL-60 cells. [234]

227. KARANDAS (Carissa carandas)
Top Recommended Edible Fruit: Karandas are very tart and mostly used to make preserves. One study of the leaf extract showed effective anticancer activity against both Caov-3 and lung cancer.[235]

228. KELP (Order: Laminariales, 30 genera)
Oceanic brown algae contain Alginates, Fucoidin, and Fucoxanthin as well as high amounts of Iodine and Vitamin K. Studies have shown that Fucoidin induces apoptosis in a wide variety of cancer cells including leukemia, colon, breast and lung cancer. Studies have also shown that Fucoxanthin dramatically reduces resistance of Prostate cancer to chemotherapy drugs. These compounds also help reduce the formation of internal blood clots that can lead to heart attack and stroke and also reduce ischemia, cholesterol levels and even help you to lose weight. [17]

229. KNOBWEED (Hyptis capitata)
Recommended Holistic Herb: Verification of the species is a must. One study isolated five triterpenoids including the new Hyptatic acid-A and -B. Hyptatic acid-A and 2α-hydroxyursolic acid showed cytotoxicity on HCT-8 cells. A study identified Oleanolic Acid and Pomolic Acid which have proven benefits as well.[236]

230. KNOTWEED (Persicaria barbata)
Recommended Holistic Herb: Verification of the species is a must because there are many species in the genus. A study found a new sesquiterpenoid which showed potent antiproliferative, pro-apoptotic, anti-metastatic and antiangiogenesis properties against: NCI-H460, MCF-7, and HeLa cell lines.[237]

231. KUDZU (Pueraria montana)
Recommended Edible Plant: A study isolated the isoflavonoids: Tectorigenin and Genistein which exhibited cytotoxicity against various cancer cell lines. Tectorigenin showed anticancer efficacy on HL-60 cells and Genistein is a known anticancer agent. [238]

232. LANGSAT (Lansium parasiticum)

Top Recommended Edible Fruit: This relative to the Lychee is similar in that it has a crust-like rind and a succulent thin layer surrounding the single hard central seed. Lychee and its relatives bring many powerful phytonutrients. One study isolated a new triterpene from the leaves. Derivatives of these compounds show significant inhibition of skin carcinogenesis. A study showed that young fruit extracts showed cytotoxicity against cancer cells. [239]

233. LAUREL FERN (Pteris ensiformis)

Top Recommended Edible Plant: Several species of fern are actually edible including this one. Young fronds are steamed and eaten like a vegetable but expert identification of the species is a must. One study identified 3 new compounds: 2R,3R-pterosin, L3-O-β-D-glucopyranoside and Pterosin B which showed cytotoxicity against HL60 cells. Another study discovered 4-Caffeoylquinic Acid 5-O-Methyl Ether and 12 other known compounds. Three compounds exhibited selective to moderate cytotoxicity.[240]

234. LAVENDER (Lavandula angustifolia)

Top Recommended Edible Plant: Many folks in the holistic medicinal circles are very familiar with Lavender Oil, but few are aware that all fresh parts of the plant above ground are edible, raw or cooked. A study of Lavender essential oil showed antimutagenic properties. [241]

235. LEICHHARDT TREE (Nauclea orientalis)

A study yielded two new alkaloid isomers, Naucleaoral A and B from the roots. Naucleaoral A showed significant cytotoxicity against HeLa cells while compound B showed modest cytotoxicity against both HeLa and KB cell lines. [242]

236. LEMON GRASS (Cymbopogon citratus)

Top Recommended Culinary Spice: Lemon grass contains several compounds in common with lemons hence its similarity in aroma and flavor, but only for occasional use since there are reports that it can have a negative impact on the liver and the brain. One study showed a-Myrcene possesses antimutagenic activity in mammary cells. The compounds, a-Limonene and Geraniol showed inhibition of liver and intestinal cancers. Another study showed inhibition of colorectal neoplasia in vivo. A study showed inhibitory effects on early phase hepatocarcinoma.[243]

237. LEOPARD LILY (Iris domestica)

A popular ornamental plant, extracts have been shown in at least one study to have anticancer powers likely linked to two phyto-estrogens: Tectorigenin and Irigenin that inhibit the proliferation of prostate cancer cells.[244]

238. LETTUCE (Lactuca sativa)

Top Recommended Superfood: Most folks think I am crazy to name Lettuce as a Superfood. But 1) it has almost no calories (3.9cal/oz), and 2) Ounce for ounce some varieties have over twice the antioxidant power of raw carrots. An aqueous extract of

49

lettuce inhibited the growth of HL-60 and MCF-7 cells. So lettuce might also help you to fight cancer too! [44]

239. LICORICE (Glycyrrhiza glabra)

Top Recommended Culinary/Holistic Herb: You would have to search hard to find true licorice any more since all confections called "Licorice" are now flavored with Anise. True licorice is powerful medicine and overindulgence is not recommended. One study yielded two new compounds and seven known phenolic compounds. Hispaglabridin B, Isoliquirtigenin, and Paratocarpin B were found to be powerful antioxidants. Isoliquirtigenin also prevented chemically-induced colon and lung tumors in vivo. A study of the root extracts showed it inhibited proliferation of HT-29 cells. [245]

240. LILAC TASSLEFLOWER (Emilia sonchifolia)

TOXIC: The plant does contain Pyrrolizidine Alkaloids that are known liver toxins. One study showed cytotoxicity and reduced the development of tumors in ascites carcinoma, lymphoma, and mouse lung fibroblast cells. Another study isolated a fraction that induced selective apoptosis in DAL. A study showed multiple selective pathways of apoptosis against HCT116. A study showed significant inhibition of lung tumor formation and metastasis. A study showed antiangiogenic effects. A study showed significant antiproliferative activity versus human cancer cells. Another study showed cytotoxicity against HeLa. Another study showed that γ-Humulene (found in many plants in the spice rack) significantly reduced cell viability through apoptosis in HT29.

241. LIMA BEAN (Phaseolus lunatus)

Top Recommended Edible Legume: Possibly the most hated of all beans: that is unfortunate because they have some amazing health benefits. They are higher in Dietary Fiber and lower in Crude Fiber than most other beans and bring a lot of Molybdenum. Studies have shown that Lima beans have a specific protein that when broken down in our digestive tract yields a substance that acts as a strong Angiotensin Converting Enzyme Inhibitor – the same kinds of compounds that are prescribed to patients suffering from chronic high blood pressure. They also possess Alpha-Amylase Inhibiting activity. This prevents the breakdown of complex sugars and starches in the digestive tract into simple sugars that can be absorbed. This means that Lima beans lower the effective calories of all of the rest of the starchy foods in the meal. Want more? Lima beans have been shown in studies to lower blood cholesterol levels, lower blood sugar levels, are hepatoprotective, protect brain cells from chemical damage, and have shown promise in stopping the growth or breast cancer. Now that should be enough to get them on the menu![459]

242. LIME (Citrus aurantifolia) *IM

Top Recommended Edible Fruit: Limes (and Lemons) are indeed sour, but they are loaded with powerful phytonutrients called Limonoids that have been shown to exhibit anticancer power and Limonoids stay in the blood much longer than most other phytonutrients, so fresh Lemonade or Limeade is a definite winner. One study of lime juice showed significant antiproliferation of human breast carcinoma cells. Another study of the oil yielded 22 compounds: D-limonene and D-dihydrocarvone being major constituents. The oil showed 78% inhibition of human colon cancer cells. Another study showed the antiproliferative effect of isolated flavonoids on AGS cancer cells.[246]

243. LOLLY FRUIT (Sandoricum koetjape)
A study isolated a new triterpenoid, Koetjapic Acid, and five known compounds and two showed significant cytotoxicity on human cancer cells. An extract showed cytotoxic and apoptotic activity against all breast cancer cell lines tested.[247]

244. LONG PEPPER (Piper retrofractum)
Top Recommended Culinary Spice: Much harder to find than Black pepper (P. nigrum) this close relative has many shared constituents including Piperine and is said to be stronger and hotter. A study of mixtures of Ginger (Z. officinale) and Long Pepper (P. retrofractum) extracts showed cytotoxicity against both HeLa and T47D cell lines.[248]

245. LOTUS (Nelumbo nucifera)
Top Recommended Holistic/Edible Plant: Lotus is another reason the Japanese are so healthy. It has a long list of beneficial properties and almost every part is edible from the rhizomes to the flowers and the plant has significant health benefits as well. One study showed the anticancer activities of N. nucifera stamen crude extract against HCT-116 cells.[249]

246. LOTUS WATER LILY (Nymphaea nouchali)
Similar in appearance to "Sacred Lotus" (Nelumbo nucifera) and also an aquatic floating species and also quite edible, one study showed marked cytotoxicity and reduced cellular invasion against B16 melanoma cells. [250]

247. LOVE GRASS (Chrysopogon aciculatus)
A study showed that Aciculatin isolated from the plant induces cell death in HCT116 in vivo.[251]

248. LYCHEE (Litchi chinensis)
Top Recommended Edible Fruit: Although expensive, it is justified; they are one of the most difficult species of fruit tree to grow and get to prosper and fruit. A study of Lychee fruit extract isolated Epicatechin, Proanthocyanidin B2 and Proanthocyanidin B4 which showed higher proliferation effects on splenocytes than the reference, Rutin. A review of Traditional Chinese Medicine treatments of human cancer notes Lychee extract could inhibit proliferation in various cancer cell lines and induce apoptosis in others. A study of Lychee fruit extract in vitro and in vivo showed it might have anticancer activity on both Estrogen Receptor positive and negative breast cancers. A study of Lychee seed extract, rich

in Polyphenols, showed significant apoptosis on two colorectal cancer cell lines.[252]

249. MADDER (Rubia cordifolia)
Recommended Edible Plant: This large leaved tall herb (to 12 feet) has more than one study showing it to have potential anticancer and cancer preventative properties. One study showed it to be effective against a human leukemia cell line while being safer toward normal human kidney cells than standard chemotherapy drugs. Another study showed a high yield extraction technique for Mollugin, a major active constituent already recognized as an anti-tumor compound against human cervical cancer.[253]

250. MAITAKE MUSHROOM (Grifola frondosa) *IM
Top Recommended Edible/Holistic Mushroom: This is another gourmet mushroom of Japanese cuisine and herbal medicine. The beta-Glucans in edible mushrooms are complex polysaccharides which have been shown in numerous studies and clinical trials to be powerful immunostimulants with strong anti-tumor activity. By the way, white Button Mushrooms (found in most grocery stores) are in this list and have beta-Glucans too.[74][254][332]

251. MALAY APPLE (Syzygium malaccense)
Top Recommended Edible Fruit: Malay Apple is likely the most well known of the Syzygium genus edible. Also known as "Rose Apple," the skin appearance is reminiscent of light colored apples though the fruit is shaped like a pear. It is an excellent low calorie fruit loaded with antioxidants and one study noted it has anticancer properties against hormone-dependent MCF-7 and non-hormone-dependent MDA-MB-231 cell lines. [255]

252. MAMEY (Pouteria sapota)
Top Recommended Edible Fruit: This tree was introduced to South Florida by the Cuban community and for good reason; the fruits are very large, and so sweet that most people prefer to cut them with ice cream or milk. Fresh Mamey is not inexpensive and difficult to come by outside of South Florida because the tree is very sensitive to temperatures near freezing that can kill it and it takes over a year for the fruits to fully ripen. A study isolated Quercetin from the fruit which exhibited anticancer properties in various tumor cell lines.[256]

253. MANGO (Mangifera indica) *IM
Top Recommended Edible Fruit: Mangoes are alone in their genus because they are actually a genetic mutation of a rare tropical fruit tree from the Bouea genus. Each cell in the Mango tree has two complete sets of the original plant's genes making their genetics quite complicated. Unpollinated flowers will yield fruits with viable seeds (that are clones of the parent) because of this curious situation. There have been extensive studies done on the fruits and they have a broad spectrum of health benefits due to the presence of powerful antioxidants as well as some fairly rare phytochemicals including Mangiferin which has been shown to

have potent anticancer properties. While all cultivated varieties bring these great health benefits, the yellow thin-skinned varieties seem to produce far less milky skin sap (a potent allergen) than the red/green skinned varieties.[45]

254. MANGOSTEEN (Garcinia mangostana)

Top Recommended Edible Fruit: Despite the name, they have absolutely nothing to do with Mangoes and are from a large genus of tropical fruit bearing bushes and trees called Garcinia and are related to another fad fruit: Gamboge (G. gamboge.) Despite the hype, Mangosteen is said to be so good that it is a contender for the "Best tasting Fruit on Earth." It does have some interesting and unique phytochemicals that in preliminary laboratory studies have shown some potent anticancer properties and I highly recommend it, but beware; with all of the recent hype about a new "miracle" fruit, there are a lot of products out there that might contain a drop or two of real Mangosteen along with a gallon from other fruits. That doesn't make them bad, but fruit punch shouldn't cost a fortune either. They adulterate the juice because Mangosteen happens to be one of THE most difficult fruit trees on Earth to cultivate to maturity and get it to fruit without dying. Many skilled botanists in South Florida have tried over the years and failed because the environmental requirements of this species are so incredibly finicky. At least ten studies have shown the plant to have significant anticancer properties against various cancer cell lines including MCF7, SK-OV-3, CEM-SS, Prostate Cancer, HCT 116, and it has shown antimutagenic properties as well. [257]

255. MARANG (Artocarpus odoratissimus)

Top Recommended Edible Fruit: Although far scarcer than its beloved kin, Jackfruit, Marang is highly prized in its native ranges of Southeast Asia, the Philippines, and through the Pacific islands. One study yielded a new flavone derivative, Artosimin, together with Traxateryl acetate. Artosimin was strongly cytotoxic against HL-60 and MCF-7.[258]

256. MARJORAM (Origanum majorana)

Top Recommended Culinary Spice: Don't underestimate the power of the culinary spices. Regular dried Marjoram that you find in the spice rack has an ORAC Score of 92,310 making it roughly 131 TIMES more potent than raw carrots. But it also brings about 40 monoterpenoids and some sesquiterpenoids, all very potent phytonutrients currently under investigation for various practical applications, and at least four preliminary studies have shown that Marjoram (a very close relative to another Top Recommended Culinary Spice – Oregano) has shown potent anticancer activity against Jurkat, Epirubicin-resistant H1299, HT-29, and MDA-MB-231. [259]

257. MARSH FLEABANE (Pluchea indica)

This plant has some unique phytonutrients that show promise in the treatment of certain types of cancer. One study yielded PITC-

2, a new compound. Synthetic derivatives similar to PITC-2 have shown cytotoxic effects against human leukemic cell lines. In another study crude aqueous root and leaf extracts suppressed proliferation, viability, and migration of HeLa and GBM8401 cells. Another study showed antiproliferative and apoptotic activity on nasopharyngeal carcinoma cells.[260]

258. MARSH MALLOW (Waltheria indica)
Unfortunately this plant has absolutely nothing to do with the tasty sugar puff confections. A study showed various leaf and stem extracts had antioxidant and cytotoxic activity against HaCaT, A549, HeLa, and HT-29.[261]

259. MILK HEDGE (Euphorbia neriifolia)
A study showed anti-tumor activity of extracts on DAL in vivo.[262]

260. MIMOSA (Mimosa pudica)
Most people have seen this plant; it is the one that reacts to being touched and folds its leaves. One study showed that Mimosine, a principle compound found in the plant, causes apoptosis and was being studied for treating ovarian cancer and other vascularized tumors. A study isolated six flavones that showed antiproliferative effects against MCF-7 and JAR.[263]

261. MIRACLE FRUIT (Synsepalum dulcificum)
Top Recommended Edible Fruit: This strange berry is growing in popularity. Alone it is basically tasteless. But after consumption of just one, everything you eat thereafter tastes better; it can even tame a terribly sour lime. This is due to a unique substance in the berry called Miraculin; basically nature's Monosodium Glutamate, but MSG is a NEUROTOXIN and Miraculin appears to be safe and therefore the only choice. It is a pet peeve of mine when I find food products still putting MSG in them like bullion cubes and even the flavor packets of some instant soups. Read those ingredient labels and if you see MSG – DON'T EAT THAT POISON; try a Miracle Fruit instead. One study showed anticancer effects against HCT-116 and HT-29.[264]

262. MULBERRY (Morus alba)
Top Recommended Edible Fruit: Dark mulberries stain the skin and definitely stain natural fibers like cotton and wool and were used by Native Americans for that purpose. However, those anthocyanidins are very powerful antioxidants and numerous studies have shown a wide array of health benefits of Mulberries including anticancer potential. And they happen to be delicious too; far better than the two close relatives that get all of the notoriety: raspberries and blackberries, both of which are Top Recommended Edible Fruits as well. At least two studies have shown anticancer efficacy against HepG2 and SW480 cells and one study has shown antimutagenic power as well.[265]

263. MULLEIN NIGHTSHADE (Solanum verbascifolium)
An excellent example of the problems with common names: this plant is not related to Mullein or the real nightshades. But it does

have a few studies suggesting that it has anticancer properties. With all species of the Solanum genus, you must get expert identification and verification of the species. While some are perfectly edible others are quite toxic and you should only use small quantities of any member of the genus to be on the safe side. Two studies showed anticancer efficacy against various cancer cell lines including LM2.[266]

264. MUSK MALLOW (Abelmoschus moschatus)
Top Recommended Holistic Herb: It has been determined that the seed oil is safe for human consumption and extracts have shown antiproliferative activity against at least two human cancer cell lines.[267]

265. MUSTARD (Brassica juncea, or B. nigrum)
Top Recommended Culinary Spice/Edible Plant: Mustard is an excellent source of sulfur compounds that the body desperately needs to build certain amino acids including those found in connective tissues like cartilage, tendons and ligaments. This close relative to Cabbage with edible leaves and seeds is loaded with antioxidants and some of those sulfur compounds have been found to have potent anticancer potential as well. Just make sure to avoid all products made yellow with artificial colors. I have found one inexpensive mustard product (name brand "Kurtz") made bright yellow with Turmeric which makes it a "double whammy" of great health benefits since Turmeric is also in this list. A study of a unique compound, Juncin, showed it has antiproliferative activity against hepatoma and breast cancer cells. A study confirmed that seed extracts (that's Mustard seed spice and the squeeze bottle products) had more anticancer efficacy than sprout extracts.[268]

266. NEEM (Azadirachta indica)
Neem is strong medicine: overindulgence is NOT recommended. A study showed the antioxidants induced apoptosis of cervical cancer cells. Another study showed a leaf extract enhanced the expression of pro-apoptotic genes.[269]

267. NICKER TREE (Caesalpinia bonducella) *IM
A study of an extract showed significant anti-tumor and antioxidant activity against EAC. Another study showed an antiproliferative and pro-apoptotic effect on EAC tumors. Another study showed 100% cytotoxicity of a stem bark extract against DAL at very low concentrations. Another study showed major anti-tumor activity against EAC in vivo. [270]

268. NIGHT BLOOMING JESSAMINE (Cestrum nocturnum)
A study isolated two new flavonoids and seven steroidal saponins. The study reports cytotoxic activities of the compounds against oral squamous cell carcinoma. Another study showed growth inhibition of tumors and prolonged life spans in vivo.[271]

269. NIPPLE FRUIT (Solanum mammosum)
Often regarded as inedible, the young fruits prior to ripening and hardening of the seeds are cooked like a vegetable. However, it is

important that the plant is properly identified as there are many species and hybrids of Solanum that are toxic to some degree and overindulgence is not recommended. One study showed efficacy against HeLa.[272]

270. NONI (Morinda citrifolia) *IM

Top Recommended Holistic Herb: Noni is legendary and while it has been the focus of quite a bit of hype in the past decade, it does have extraordinary holistic properties. Overindulgence is not recommended. A study notes the prevention of chemically induced DNA damage and the antioxidant activity from commercial juice may contribute to the cancer preventive effect. A study showed a growth inhibitory effect on cancer. Two independent studies found that leaf extracts were better than the approved anticancer drug Erlotinib; one showed this effect against lung adenocarcinoma, the other showed its anticancer potency against A549 cells in vitro and NSCLC in vivo. [273]

271. NORFOLK PINE (Araucaria heterophylla)

Did you know that the resin of a Christmas tree might be able to cure cancer? Studies have verified that the plant is relatively non-toxic as well. One study demonstrated anticancer efficacy against both MCF7 and HCT116 cell lines.[274]

272. NUT GRASS (Cyperus rotundus)

Recommended (Limited dosage): Nut Grass is considered to be the #1 Invasive Weed on Earth and it is found virtually everywhere. It could be in the nearest empty lot from where you are right now. For a hated weed, the plant packs a punch in antioxidant power and several interesting and unique phytonutrients as well. Despite the long list of potential health benefits, very little study has been done on the plant concerning human health and safety (most work involves how to kill it!) and caution is advised. A study showed it has anticancer efficacy against EAC.[275]

273. OKRA (Abelmoschus esculentus)

Top Recommended Edible Fruit: Like many other fruits most people consider Okra to be a vegetable and that's fine since "Vegetable" is not a scientific term. Most people don't like Okra because of its "sliminess" which is the high mucilage content in the seed pods, but sliced and fried in corn meal breading they are excellent (despite the frying and the corn meal breading which are both Top Foods to Avoid.) However, the goal is to find a way to turn the evil foods into good ones and Fried Okra might be one of the few acceptable fried, breaded, foods. Two studies showed efficacy against MCF-7 and B16F10 cells.[50]

274. OLIVES (Olea europea)

Top Recommended Superfood: Olives are high in Oleuropein found in trace amounts in a study of Globe Amaranth to have broad spectrum anticancer power. The other major compounds in olives are Tyrosol, Hydroxytyrosol, Demethyloleuropein, Oleanolic Acid, Erythrodiol, Elenoic Acid, Ligstroside, Apigenin, Luteolin,

Caffeic Acid, Cinnamic Acid, Ferulic Acid, Coumaric Acid, Uvaol, Anthocyanidins, Quercetin, Vanillic Acid, Gallic Acid, Kaempferol, Protocatechuic Acid, and Syringic Acid. Many of these compounds have studies showing potent anticancer power. Extra Virgin Oil is loaded with these compounds and home made Oil and Vinegar dressing should be the ONLY thing that goes on your salad.[46]

275. ONION (Allium cepa)

Top Recommended Edible Plant: Onions, preferably cooked, are a rich source of glucosinolates like their relatives, Garlic, Leeks and Shallots (also in this list.) Onions have shown neuroprotective, gastroprotective, nephroprotective, hypotensive and hypolipidemic properties and efficacy against multidrug resistant erythroleukemia and K562 cancer cell lines. Overindulgence in raw onions could have a negative effect on red blood cells; so cook 'em up.[51]

276. ORANGE CLIMBER (Toddalia asiatica)

Recommended Edible Fruit: Expert identification of this vine is a must because they are rarely seen and could resemble any of hundreds of poisonous species of fruiting vines. The small berries born in rows along the branch tips are said to taste like a cross between orange and lemon. The plant possesses some unique phytochemicals that have been shown to selectively target and kill various types of cancer cells. One study isolated 3 new unusual compounds: DHN (Dihydronitidine) NTD (Nitidine), and DMN (Demthylnitidine). NTD and DHN selectively inhibited growth of human lung adenocarcinoma in vitro. Another study showed leaf oil has considerable antioxidant potency and protects the DNA of human lymphocytes and is cytotoxic to MCF-7 and HT-29.[276]

277. ORCHID TREE (Bauhinia variegata) *IM

Recommended Edible Plant: Not many people know that this popular widespread ornamental tree's displays of pink/lavender orchid-like flowers are actually edible, although it is usually the unopened buds that are cooked like a vegetable. There are over 200 species of Bauhinia and many have impressive medicinal properties including this one. Bark extracts have been shown to have possible anticancer, antimutagenic and chemoprotective properties against skin papilloma, DU-145, HOP-62, IGR-OV-1, MCF-7, THP-1, malignant HeLa and B16F10 cell lines. The extracts used in most studies were shown to be non-toxic. Orchid Tree has one of the widest ranges of cancers it can fight in this list and that has also been determined to be relatively safe.[277]

278. OREGANO (Origanum vulgare)

Top Recommended Culinary Spice: Oregano has one of the highest ORAC Scores of any widely available edible product at 175,295. That means that Oregano has about 250 TIMES the antioxidant power of raw carrots. Just 4 grams of dried Oregano leaves available at just about any grocery store has the antioxidant potency of over 2 POUNDS of RAW CARROTS. Add that heaping teaspoon to soups, stews, casseroles, tomato sauce and Oil and

Vinegar dressing and you have made them all into very powerful foods. But the benefits are only just beginning; Oregano has a host of powerful phytonutrients with many health benefits including the potential to help defeat cancer including MCF-7 and HeLa.[278]

279. OTAHEITE GOOSEBERRY (Phyllanthus acidus)

Top Recommended Edible Fruit: Not at the top of very many lists as an edible fruit, Otaheite Gooseberry is quite sour and mostly made into preserves. The leaves can be cooked like a vegetable and there are several studies showing it has anticancer power. Stay away from the roots though, they are toxic. A study showed significant in vitro cytotoxicity against HepG2 and DAL cell lines. A study of an extract showed significant anticancer effect on both MCF-7 and SSC-40.[279]

280. OYSTER MUSHROOM (Pleurotus spp.) *IM

Top Recommended Edible Mushroom: All edible mushrooms (in this list) bring powerful phytonutrients called beta-Glucans which have been shown to provide significant immune boosting power as well as amazing anticancer properties. While store bought Button or Portabella mushrooms do bring these important beta-Glucans, the gourmet mushrooms bring far more and each species has a different array of beta-Glucans which can have a significant impact on their potency and specific health benefits and they all come highly recommended.[74][332]

281. PAPAYA (Carica papaya) *IM

Top Recommended Edible Fruit: Being loaded with antioxidants and flavonoids as well as Papain make the fruit, not only delicious but also a great benefit for health including: gastroprotective, and hepatoprotective (better than megadosing on Vitamin E, which can be dangerous.) One study showed efficacy against 10 different cancers including cervical, breast, liver, lung, and pancreatic cell lines. Another study showed anticancer efficacy on K562. A study showed significant inhibition of both MCF-7 and MDA-MB-231. Another showed selective cytotoxicity against MDA-MB-231, AGS, HL-60, MCF-7, T47D, and squamous carcinoma, amongst many others. [47]

282. PARSLEY (Petroselinum crispum)

Top Recommended Culinary Spice: Although it does contain oxalates which are both irritants and toxic, we don't consume nearly enough to be a problem especially if it is cooked thoroughly in soups and stews which dissolve and break up oxalates in the boiling in water and the U.S. has classified it as GRAS – Generally Recognized As Safe. In the meantime, Parsley brings antioxidants and other phytonutrients that make significant contributions to human health and may help fight cancer including HepG2 and MCF-7. [280]

283. PASSION FRUIT (Passiflora edulis)

Top Recommended Edible Fruit: Passiflora is a confusing genus of deciduous vines many of which yield edible fruits. It is confusing because some experts suspect that most of the identified species may in fact be fertile natural hybrids and even P. edulis has two varieties, Yellow Lillikoi and Purple Lillikoi. The purple one is suspected of containing toxic phytochemicals but it is the Yellow Lillikoi that is used in the production of most commercial fruit juices anyway. There is mounting evidence that this fruit's unique and powerful antioxidants and flavonoids provide a broad spectrum of health benefits including anticancer properties. One study showed its anticancer efficacy against CCRF-CEM and drug resistant CEM-ADR5000 cells.[281]

284. PASTUREWEED (Cyathula prostrata)
A study showed high activity against HeLa. Another study showed cytotoxicity against HeLa and U937 cell lines. A study showed anti-tumor and antioxidant properties against DAL cells in vivo. Another study showed the anticancer activity of an extract against EAC in vivo. Another study showed anticancer activity by induction of cell cycle arrest through an unknown mechanism. Another study showed cytotoxicity against the HeLa cell line.[282]

285. PATCHOULI (Pogostemon cablin)
Patchouli oil derived from this plant is very popular in Indian Ayurvedic medicine, Traditional Chinese Medicine, and it is also used in cosmetics. Very small doses are allowed in food (up to 0.0002%) and limited usage of the oil (one milliliter/gal) is roughly this concentration. One study of an extract suppressed the effects of the mutagen furylfuramide and isolated suppressive compounds like 7,4'-di-O-methyleriodictyol, Pachypodol, Kumatekenin and Mobuine.[283]

286. PAU D'ARCO (Tabebuia spp.) *IM
Top Recommended Holistic Herb: Many species of Tabebuia are popular as ornamental landscaping trees because of their showy flowers, but the inner bark tea has been shown to ward off many infections and help prevent many nasty tropical diseases including Malaria. Studies have shown it is effective in protecting the stomach and liver and it has shown anticancer properties.[284]

287. PEACOCK MOSS (Selaginella uncinata)
Recommended (Limited): Neither a moss nor much of a "Peacock" this unassuming little herb may turn out to have anticancer power. One study showed efficacy against HT-29. [285]

288. PEANUT (Arachis hypogaea)
Top Recommended Edible Seed/Nut: While Sunflower seeds are the #1 seed/nut in terms of the number of nutrients and the amounts they bring, Peanuts are no slouches by any means. A 3 oz. serving brings 21% of your daily fiber requirement and a third of your daily Magnesium requirement (a mineral that is difficult to get in 100% RDA amounts from natural whole foods on a daily basis.) One study showed that the unique phytonutrients found in peanuts might help fight cancer so they have a lot going for them. Just watch those calories even though they are due to very healthy

monounsaturated fats and monounsaturated fatty acids (MUFAs) they are still very fattening if you are not careful. And don't forget that ORAC score of 3432, they have about 5 times the antioxidant potency of an equal weight of raw carrots. Another study found that PNA showed significant cytotoxicity toward the human cancer cell lines HeLa and Hep-2.[1]

289. PEARL GRASS (Oldenlandia corymbosa)

A study showed promising results as an antitumor agent against implanted malignant tumors and protective effect against radiation-induced hematopoeitic damage. Another study of the components: Ursolic Acid, Oleanolic Acid, and Geniposidic Acid showed the first two inhibited the growth of Hep2B cells. Extracts showed potential anticancer activity with growth inhibitory activity to YMB-1. Another study showed anticarcinogenic properties of the combined extracts of Soursop (Annona muricata) and Pearl Grass. Another study of a leaf extract showed significant anticancer activity against K562. A study of an extract showed anticancer power against MMP-9.[286]

290. PERIWINKLE (Vinca rosea)

TOXIC: This is the ubiquitous and easily grown flower found in most well stocked garden centers. Two alkaloids have been isolated from Vinca for use as approved anticancer drugs: Vincristine and Vinblastine. But, toxicity from the leaves can creep up quickly and once it appears, it continues to progress (even after ceasing consumption) and can be FATAL. I include the plant here for the warning, and to illustrate the fact that some plants have already provided us with approved chemotherapy drugs. Vinca is NOT RECOMMENDED for home use.[287]

291. PHILIPPINE ALMOND (Terminalia calamansanai)

This close relative of the Tropical almond (T. catappa) and Black Myrobalan (T. chebula) has some interesting compounds called ellagitannins found in the leaf extract that show promise in the treatment and prevention of certain forms of cancer. In one study 2-O-Galloylpunicalin and Sanguiin H-4 found in an extract of the leaves inhibited the viability of HL-60 cells.[288]

292. PHILIPPINE CEDAR (Toona calantas)

One study yielded a compound with significant cytotoxicity and mild to moderate anti-tumor activity.[289]

293. PIGEON PEA (Cajanus cajan)

Top Recommended Edible Legume: This pea is unusual in that it is produced by shrub rather than a small herb like most others. Cajanol, an isoflavanone, isolated from the roots, inhibited growth of MCF-7 cells via apoptosis.[290]

294. PILI NUT (Canarium ovatum)

A study showed promising antimutagenic activity by reducing the number of damaged red blood cells by greater than 50%.[291]

295. PINEAPPLE (Ananas comosus)

Top Recommended Edible Fruit: Pineapple and its principle phytonutrient, Bromelain, have been linked to aiding digestion and also show powerful anti-diabetic potential. Bromelain has been linked in at least one study to having anti-tumor properties as well making Pineapple a very healthy fruit that should be included in everyone's diet.[54]

296. PINECONE GINGER (Zingiber zerumbet)

This close relative to the real ginger has a phytochemical called Zerumbone which in three independent studies showed powerful anticancer effectiveness against P-388D1, HepG2, MCF-7, and HL-60.[292]

297. PINK WAMPEE (Clausena excavata)

Top Recommended Edible Fruit: There are two members of the Clausena genus in this list and most people have never seen or heard of them, but they are related to citrus. One study of Clausine B, an alkaloid isolated from the stem bark, showed activity against non-hormone-dependent breast cancer, cervical cancer, ovarian cancer and hepatic cancer. Another study showed the fruit extract had cytotoxic activity against MCF-7 cells. Another study yielded four unique compounds: Clausenidin, Nordentatin, Clausarin and Xanthoxyletin. Two showed cytotoxicity against four human cancer cell lines. Others showed significant activity against multi-drug resistant cancer cell lines. Another study showed that an extract inhibited HeLa cell proliferation by 50%. Another study showed the antiproliferative potential of Dentatin, a coumarin from C. excavata, against prostate cancer cell lines. Another study yielded six coumarins and twelve alkaloids from the roots. Three had high cytotoxicity against KB, MCF-7, and NCI-H187. Another study showed significant reduction in tumor volume of tumors induced in LA-7 cells in vivo. [293]

298. POLYANTHUS LILY (Polianthes tuberosa)

Recommended Edible Flowers: Another of the few species of edible lily, Polyanthus is a very popular ornamental for its showy white flowers and strong lovely aroma. Natives cook those flowers into soups and stews and they have verified health benefits, just be absolutely certain that you have the correct species because many species of lilies are POISONOUS. A study isolated a new glycoside and 3 new saponins along with a known glycoside. The compounds were cytotoxic toward HL-60.[294]

299. POMEGRANATE (Punica granatum) *IM

Top Recommended Edible Fruit: Pomegranate fruit and juice has a very high ORAC score and it is loaded with many unique phytonutrients including Punicic Acid. One study showed that the extracts of juice, seed oil and peel significantly inhibited prostate cancer cell invasiveness, proliferation, and induced cell death and inhibited tumor growth. Another study showed similar anticancer power against the PC3 cell line. Another study showed inhibition of cell proliferation in MV4-11 and K562 cells via apoptosis. A study noted that the ellagitannins and urolithins liberated in the colon from the juice in considerable amounts could slow colon cancer progress through inhibition of cell proliferation and induction of apoptosis. Another study showed breast cancer preventative potential for the purified juice and seed oil.[56]

300. POMELO (Citrus maxima)
Top Recommended Edible Fruit: While not as well known or available as its hybrid offshoot, Grapefruit, Pomelo and Grapefruit share similar phytochemistry including interactions with metabolic enzymes that encourage weight-loss, lower blood pressure, blood sugar, and blood cholesterol levels. Analysis of fruit extract yielded 76 compounds. Limonene prevailed as well as a-Terpineol, (E,E)-2,4-Decadienal, Hexadecanoic Acid, Pentacosane, Stigmasterol, and gamma-Sitosterol. The fruit extracts showed antiproliferative effects toward human brain glioblastoma, gastric cancer, cervical adenocarcinoma and gastric adenocarcinoma.[3]

301. POPPING POD (Ruellia tuberosa)
One of many different and unrelated species that have seed pods that burst open (this one when it gets wet) and fling the seeds out. At least three studies have shown anticancer efficacy against MCF-7, HepG2, and EAC.[295]

302. PORTABELLA MUSHROOM (Agaricus bisporus) *IM
Top Recommended Edible Mushroom: See Button Mushroom.

303. PORTIA TREE (Thespesia populnea)
A close relative to the Hibiscus and often placed in its genus; one study showed a decoction of T. populnea and Adenanthera pavonina had antiproliferative activity and induced apoptosis on Hep-2 cancer cells.[296]

304. POTATO BUSH (Phyllanthus reticulatus)
One study showed anticancer properties against HT-29. [297]

305. POUZOLZS BUSH (Pouzolzia zeylanica)
A study showed cytotoxicity and suggested a promising source for anticancer compounds. [298]

306. PRICKLY ASH (Zanthoxylum avicennae)
One study showed dose-dependent induction of apoptosis on HA22T cells in vitro and in vivo. [299]

307. PRICKLY POPPY (Argemone mexicana)
One study showed the cytotoxicity of alkaloids from this plant on SW480. Jatrorrhizine and 8-Methoxydihydrosanguinarine showed the highest potency of inhibiting cancer cell proliferation (95 to 100%) showing complete reduction of cell viability. This is one of the more exciting results in this entire list.[300]

308. PUMPKIN (Cucurbita maxima)
Top Recommended Edible Fruit: Although flower, leaf and seed extracts were evaluated for their anticancer potential, pumpkin fruit and roasted seeds are highly nutritious and highly recommended. One study showed anticancer activity via apoptosis of compounds isolated from the flowers against HepG2. Another study of a seed extract yielded Demosterol which showed high binding affinity to androgen cell receptors and may have anticancer potential.[57]

309. PURPLE TEPHROSIA (Tephrosia purpurea)
A study showed a root extract has potent chemoprotective efficacy and significant reduction of lipid peroxidation in DMBA-induced oral carcinogenesis. Another study showed significant anti-tumor activity in DEN-induced liver cancer in vivo. Another study showed anticancer potential against MCF-7. A study showed anticancer effect of root extracts against EAC cell lines in vivo comparable to the standard drug 5-FU. [301]

310. PURSLANE (Portulaca oleracea)
Top Recommended Edible Plant: Don't be fooled by the small dark spaghetti-like stems, sparse leaves and pretty flowers of this very common garden flower. The above ground parts are all edible and fresh leaves are excellent in salads. It has been shown to be a nephroprotective plant despite having oxalate crystals in it. A small amount of leaves added to a salad, or made into a decoction herbal tea (better since boiling water neutralizes oxalates) once a week should be safe. One study of an aqueous extract showed tumoricidal activity against human gastric and human colon cancer cell lines. A study showed significant reduction in tumor volume and inhibition of tumor growth of mammary adenocarcinoma in vivo with extensive tumor cell necrosis and no general toxicity of the extract. Another study showed significant reduction of cell viability of HepG2 and A549 cell lines using seed oil. A study showed antiproliferative and cytotoxic effect against HT-29, HeLa, CNE-1 and hormone-dependent MCF-7. [302]

311. PUZZLENUT TREE (Xylocarpus granatum)
One study isolated Xylogranin B which showed strong cytotoxicity against colon cancer cell lines. [303]

312. QUASSIA (Quassia indica)
Prolonged usage can cause Kidney and Liver damage: Bark extracts have been used as topical treatments for skin infections and arthritis. The plant contains a group of unique compounds called Quassinoids have been shown to have anti-inflammatory, antiviral and anti-tumor properties.[410]

313. RADISH (Raphanus sativus)
Top Recommended Edible Plant: While radishes are well known for their edible rhizomes, all parts of the plant are edible. With hundreds of hybrids and varieties, it is difficult to pin down which ones are the most effective, but sliced raw in salads or cooked as a vegetable they are very low in calories, high in copper, and at least one study has shown that they do possess some power to kill certain types of colon cancer, but don't overdo it, excessive copper can become toxic. One study showed that a polysaccharide in radishes, Galactan, has pronounced cytotoxic effects on colon cancer cell lines.[304]

314. RAMBUTAN (Nephelium lappaceum)
Top Recommended Edible Fruit: A relative to the lychee, this bright red fruit looks like a sea urchin except that the long thin

bright red spines are rubbery and harmless. Inside it is a large seed surrounded by a thin white layer of pulp that is similar to lychee. Most of the experimentation showing antioxidant and anticancer power and has been done with extract of the unusual rind and not the fruit, but the fruit is edible and worth a try.[305]

315. RED CLOVER (Trifolium pratense)
Top Recommended Holistic Herb: Use this one in moderation as it has many warnings of being poisonous in excess. Red Clover is loaded with phytoestrogens and considered effective in easing women's hormonal issues. It has also been shown to have efficacy against certain breast cancer cell lines.[306]

316. RED COTTON (Asclepias curassavica) *IM
Calotropin in the extract of this plant showed cytotoxicity against human nasopharyngeal carcinoma cells. Another study isolated unique compounds from A. curassavica and most of them showed pronounced cytotoxicity against four different cancer cell lines. Beta-Sitosterol has been shown in many studies to significantly inhibit growth of colon cancer. A study evaluated 10 medicinal herbs used in India as treatments for cancer: all 10 showed significant antioxidant and antiproliferative activities with A. curassavica showing the highest activity. Another study found Asclepin which showed the strongest cytotoxic activity against HepG2 and Raji cells. Another study identified a novel glycoside, asclepiasterol, capable of reversing P-gp-mediated multidrug resistance by enhancing the cytotoxicity of anticancer drugs against MCF-7/ADR and HepG2/ADM cells.[307]

317. RED GINGER (Alpinia purpurata)
One study showed this close relative to true ginger has anticancer efficacy against PA1. Another study showed anticancer efficacy against HeLa. [308]

318. RED SORREL (Hibiscus sabdariffa)
Top Recommended Holistic Herb: Also marketed as Hibiscus Tea, this is one of the most powerful hypotensive herbs on the market. It is so effective at lowering blood pressure that it should be taken in very low doses and never in combination with any other blood pressure lowering medications or herbs. Loaded with anthocyanidins it has also been shown to have a powerful effect against MCF-7 and non-cancerous MCF12A breast cell lines.[309]

319. RED TREE VINE (Leea guinensis)
This is another unassuming species of Leea, small vines or shrubs yielding branched bunches of berries. The healing powers are in the leaves, bark and roots. A study showed that extracts are non-toxic and have significant antioxidant and antitumor effects.[310]

320. REISHI MUSHROOM (Ganoderma lucidum) *IM
Top Recommended Edible Mushroom: Its name means "Spirit" in Japanese and with a traditional herbal medicinal history going back centuries in China and Japan, Reishi mushroom is very well known for being a potent tonic for longevity and vitality as well as

being effective against hepatitis and cirrhosis of the liver due to alcohol abuse. Its power is believed to be in the immunostimulant properties of its high concentrations of beta-Glucans, unusual polysaccharides found in high concentrations in certain edible mushrooms. Beta-Glucans have also been shown to have potent anti-tumor activity as well. Many of these edible mushrooms have always been considered powerful medicine and gourmet foods making them expensive, but now that the science backs up their claims they have become very expensive. However, even Button mushrooms found in most grocery stores have plenty of beta-Glucans too, but at a fraction of the price. [74][311][332]

321. RESURRECTION PLANT (Bryophyllum pinnatum)
This unusual plant develops seedlings along the notches of its leaves which grow until they fall off and in favorable conditions will continue to grow up into an adult plant. Such seedlings are clones of the parent which can produce flowers and seeds normally as well. Due to its POTENTIAL TOXICITY usage is not recommended despite a long list of holistic medicinal properties including studies showing its effectiveness against some forms of cancer.[312]

322. RIBBON PLANT (Chlorophytum comosum)
One study showed anticancer efficacy against HeLa, CCRF-HSB-2, HL-60 and U937 cell lines.[313]

323. ROOIBOS (Aspalathus linearis) *IM
Top Recommended Holistic Herb: Rooibos is considered to be one of the safest medicinal herbs in this list with no reported toxicity or negative side effects in centuries of use. Also called "Redbush tea" because of the bright red leaves, they actually turn red during the sun drying process as a natural result of the action of certain enzymes. The tea is loaded with antioxidants and it is considered an immunostimulant and anticancer agent.[314]

324. ROSE (Rosa spp. and hybrids)
Top Recommended Holistic Herb: Roses and Rose hips (the swollen base of the flower that is filled with seeds) are very well known in holistic medicinal circles. There are potentially hundreds of species and thousands of hybrids and cultivars but one in particular, R. canina blossoms and rose hips, has shown a very potent effect inhibiting A-172, U-251 MG, and U-1231 MG with greater effect than the approved drug Temozolomide.[315]

325. ROSE LEADWORT (Plumbago indica)
An in vivo study showed a close relative to have a weak anti-tumor effect, but it enhanced the tumor-killing effect of radiation therapy. Another study showed the anti-tumor and radiation-modifying properties of Plumbagin in vivo against EAC. Another study showed Plumbagin inhibited tumor growth. All Plumbagos should be considered TOO TOXIC FOR HOME USE.[316]

326. ROSEMARY (Rosmarinus officinalis) *IM
Top Recommended Culinary Spice: Both major components, Carnosol and Rosmarinic Acid have been shown in preliminary

laboratory investigations to have significant anticancer properties. Rosemary also shows pathways of action in the brain that may indicate some effectiveness in the treatment of Alzheimer's disease and improvement of cognitive function. Rosemary is a powerful double whammy; it's brain food and fights cancer. [317]

327. ROYAL POINCIANA (Delonix regia)

Top Recommended Holistic Herb: Royal Poinciana trees are truly majestic. They can become huge and covered in fiery orange flowers in full bloom. A study showed potent anticancer effect against HepG2. Another study of the flower extract showed anticancer effects against: MCF-7, HeLa, brain carcinoma, and colon carcinoma cell lines.[318]

328. RUBBER PLANT (Ficus elastica)

Another very well known member of the Ficus genus, but the plant is TOXIC and interest is mostly scientific and USAGE OF THE PLANT IS NOT RECOMMENDED. One study showed antioxidant activity possibly due to its rich polyphenolic content and flavonoids. Fractions showed activity against liver and breast human tumor cell lines.[319]

329. SACRED FIG TREE (Ficus religiosa)

Ficus is a vast genus of plants with well over 200 species. Within those many species there are Top Recommended Edible Fruits like the Fig (F. carica) as well as toxic species. This one does not appear to be so toxic or allergenic and it is the bark that seems to have most of the holistic properties. Just make sure that your source has correctly identified the species and is not making a substitution with one of the hundreds of other species of Ficus. A study reported the antineoplastic potential of the aqueous extract on HeLa cell lines via induced apoptosis. Another study showed cytotoxicity on PC3-TxR cells resistant to Docetaxel in vitro. [320]

330. SAFFLOWER (Carthamus tinctorius)

Top Recommended Holistic Herb: Not that Safflower Oil will cure cancer, but extracts of the flowers and leaves have shown strong anticancer properties in more than one study. One study of Zhyu-xiang extracts containing Ginseng and C. tinctorius, showed significant inhibition in cell proliferation against the MDA-MB-231 cell line. Another study showed immunostimulant activity. Another study of an extract on dendritic cell vaccine showed a dramatic increase in levels of TNF-α and IL-1ß, with great immunological and co-stimulatory activity. Another study showed inhibition of proliferation and metastasis of MCF-7.[321]

331. SAGE (Salvia officinalis)

Top Recommended Culinary Spice: Many common spices found in the baking isle of your grocery store are very powerful medicine; Sage is one of them. It contains Perillyl Alcohol which has been found to inhibit harmful factors in the brain meaning it is a powerful neuroprotective and nootropic (increases cognitive brain function, memory, mood, clarity, etc.) It has also been shown to have potent anticancer properties, but it may antagonize liver toxins (it is not a liver toxin itself, but it may boost the effects of other liver toxins, i.e. alcohol.) and moderation is advised.[322]

332. SANDPAPER TREE (Streblus asper)

The leaves are used as a substitute for sandpaper. One study found that the major constituents of the leaf oil were Phytol, A-Farnesene, Trans-Farnesyl Acetate, Caryophyllene and Trans-Trans-A-Farnesene. This oil showed significant cytotoxicity on leukemia lymphocytes. Another study showed root extract caused cell death in osteosarcoma cells. A study showed an extract had anti-tumor and antioxidant effect against EAC in vivo. Plants like this with anticancer activity against bone cancers are RARE.[323]

333. SAPPAN WOOD (Caesalpinia sappan)

Top Recommended Holistic Herb: Sappan is a large tree and the heartwood is the richest source of Brazilin which has a whole list of positive health benefits because it is a powerful antioxidant. One such benefit is that it has shown strong inhibition of many different cancer cell lines including HeLa, HNSCC4, HNSCC31 ovarian cancer, A549, and breast cancer.[324]

334. SCREW PINE (Pandanus tectorius)

A study of an extract of stem bark showed strong cytotoxicity on the KB cell line. A study isolated: Stigmast-4-en-3-one, Stimasta-4,22-dien-3-one, Cycloucalenol, and Stigmast-22-en-3ß-ol. The second compound showed cytotoxicity against KB.[325]

335. SEA ROSEMALLOW (Hibiscus tiliaceus) *IM

Yet another species of Hibiscus in this list; they all have strong medicinal power and overindulgence is not recommended. At least three studies show this species has anticancer efficacy against DAL, as well as both antigenotoxic and antimutagenic effects that protect against oxidative DNA damage.[326]

336. SEASIDE PLUM (Ximenia americana)

Top Recommended Edible Fruit: Only a tiny fraction of 1% of all plants produce edible parts. Ximenia is one of them and not many people have ever seen them. Overindulgence of fully tree ripened fruit is not recommended (true of most edible fruits by the way, they turn purgative in a hurry.) One study isolated a new protein, Riproximin, a Type II RIP that showed significant inhibition of colorectal cancer metastasis. Another study showed significant antineoplastic (95% reduction) activity.[327]

337. SEPTIC FIG (Ficus septica)

A study yielded Phenanthroindolizidine N-oxide, Ficuseptine-A together with 18 known compounds from the leaves. Some of the compounds exhibited strong cytotoxic activity against two human cancer cell lines. Another study showed a leaf extract has potential as a chemoprotective combined with Doxorubicin. Another study of the leaf extract showed anticancer efficacy inducing apoptosis in liver cancer. Another study showed positive effects of a leaf extract in combination with Doxorubicin on cytotoxicity, cell cycle arrest, and apoptosis against T47D. [328]

338. SESAME (Sesamum indicum)

Top Recommended Edible Seed: The best way to consume sesame seed is in the form of sesame seed butter, a product called "Tahini." Aside from noted anticancer potential, sesame seed also increases the levels of potassium in the blood while lowering the levels of Sodium and is suspected of being a major influence in the reduction of high blood pressure and the risk for cardiovascular disease. One study showed inhibition of: Hep-2, AMN-3, and RD cell lines.[60]

339. SHAGGY BUTTON WEED (Spermacoce hispida)

Recommended Edible Plant: The whole small weed is edible, cooked as a vegetable, and it has shown anticancer activity in at least two studies; one against A549 and HeLa cancer cells, and the other against PA-1.[329]

340. SHALLOT (Allium ascalonicum)

Top Recommended Edible Plant: Chinese Red Onions are excellent for your health and might help fight cancer too. One study showed an aqueous extract had the most growth inhibition activity on the cancer cell lines tested. Another study showed both dry and fresh shallot extracts exhibited anticancer properties.[330]

341. SHIITAKE MUSHROOM (Lentinus edodes) *IM

Top Recommended Edible Mushroom: This is another gourmet mushroom featuring the powerful immunostimulant and anticancer beta-Glucans. Not all beta-Glucans are the same and most of these gourmet mushrooms have much more beta-Glucans than Button or Portabella mushrooms (also in this list.) They are more expensive, but the different forms of Beta-Glucans found in the gourmet mushrooms may have greater medicinal powers.[74][332]

342. SHINY BUSH (Peperomia pellucida)

Recommended Edible Plant: The leaves and young stems are treated like a vegetable and studies have confirmed that this plant is safe and has potential anticancer properties as well.[331]

343. SHOOFLY (Caesalpinia decapetala)

One study isolated Emodin, Baicalein, and Apigenin which showed significant anti-tumor activities against the MGC-803 cell line. [333]

344. SICKLEPOD (Senna tora)

Normally I would recommend a safe and strong anticancer plant, but the Senna, Cassia and Acacia genera are all related and contain hundreds of species of trees that are often confused or purposely substituted making it difficult to verify the plant or the content of any product claiming to use it. One study showed that the extract induced a marked inhibition of proliferation, reduced DNA content, and induced apoptosis in HeLa. A study showed anticancer activity against MCF-7. A study showed anticancer effects in TCA8113d cells by significant induction of apoptosis, and also had anti-inflammatory activity and exerted an anti-metastatic effect in vivo.[334]

345. SINGAPORE RHODODENDRON (Melastoma malabathricum)
Recommended Edible Fruit: The leaves of the plant are also edible when cooked. Three studies showed anticancer efficacy against: DAL, HepG2, and MCF-7 cell lines.[335]

346. SLENDER CARPETWEED (Glinus oppositifolius)
Due to the presence of several strong antioxidants it has been shown to have anti-proliferative properties on more than one human cancer cell line.[336]

347. SMARTWEED (Persicaria hydropiper)
Recommended Edible Plant: Leaves and stems are edible raw or cooked however, expert verification of the species is a must. One study showed anti-tumor cytotoxicity.[337]

348. SNAKE GOURD (Trichosanthes cucumerina)
Recommended Edible Fruit: Another Cucurbit or member of the vine-borne melons, this one has a bit of a laxative effect and is not nearly as popular as most other well known species. One study found 13 compounds in the plant have already been shown to inhibit prostate cancer progression. Two other studies showed anticancer efficacy of Cucurbitacin B against SKBR-3, MCF-7, HBL-100, T47D and colon cancer.[338]

349. SNAKE NEEDLE GRASS (Oldenlandia diffusa)
Recommended Holistic Herb: There are many preliminary studies with this herb focusing on its measurable anticancer effects on a wide variety of human cancer cell lines and it is one of the few that might be successful in human clinical trials. Two species are often used interchangeably although O. corymbosa (Pearl Grass, also in this list) is higher in Oleanolic and Ursolic Acid which is believed to be a major contributing factor to its medicinal potential.[339]

350. SNAKE WEED (Euphorbia hirta)
Recommended Holistic Herb: Not the most inviting name, but it does come from old medicinal usage to treat snake bite victims and there is scientific evidence that it does neutralize the venom of some species of poisonous snakes. It has also been shown to be an effective treatment for asthma and numerous studies have also shown that it could also turn out to be a very potent anticancer treatment. One study showed extracts have selective cytotoxicity on several cancer cell lines. Leaf extract showed anti-proliferative activity on Hep-2. Another study showed anti-tumor activity on EL-4 in vivo. Another study showed anticancer effects against DAL and EAC.[340]

351. SNEEZE WEED (Centipeda minima)
A fraction showed broad spectrum inhibitory effects on five human cancer cell lines: MCF-7, PC-3, HepG2, CNE, and HL-60. Another study showed significant inhibition of proliferation against CNE-1. A study showed the pathway of action of 6-O-Angeloylplenolin, a terpenoid that induces apoptosis in human multiple myeloma.[341]

352. SOUR ORANGE (Citrus x aurantium)

Top Recommended Edible Fruit: There are plenty of weight-loss products based on Citrus, usually Sour Orange (or Bitter Orange) and like Pomelo (and Grapefruit, also in this list) they do possess compounds that stimulate fat burning metabolism and there is a concern that these products contain too much Synephrine (similar in effects to the banned Ephedrine) which can cause increased heart rate and elevated blood pressure. Eating fully tree ripened fruit is always far safer than taking the refined supplements. One study showed the anticancer effects of isolated flavonoids against AGS cells. Another study showed cytotoxicity of the essential oil on a colorectal cancer cell line. Limonene and Myrcene are the main components.]342]

353. SOURSOP (Annona muricata)

Top Recommended Edible Fruit: One of160+ species of Annona trees most of which produce edible fruit and Soursop like many of the others is quite large, odd-looking (looks like a 2 pound bright green kidney been covered in harmless rubbery thorns) and exquisite. Soursop has been in the news as numerous studies have shown that it does have a measurable anticancer effect. Although most studies are using leaf, bark and root extracts, the fruit also contains some of the active compounds. Herbal teas from the leaves are far more potent. However, EXCESSIVE usage of Soursop can lead to KIDNEY PROBLEMS. For those who wish to pursue this plant's anticancer powers, drink plenty of water and pursue other holistic herbs with nephroprotective properties. One study showed that one of the acetogenins was selectively cytotoxic to colon adenocarcinoma cells, with a potency 10,000 TIMES that of the approved anticancer drug Adriamycin. A study showed extracts to be effective against growth of Adriamycin-resistant MCF-7/Adr. Analysis of fruit flesh yielded cis-Annoreticuin which showed cytotoxicity against HepG2. A study showed Acetogenin 1 was cytotoxic on PACA-2, PC-3 and A549. A study of leaf extract showed antiproliferative effects on BPH-1 with reduced prostate size, possibly through apoptosis. In another study seeds yielded seven new acetogenins: Muricin A to G, together with five known compounds. The acetogenins showed significant selective in vitro cytotoxicity toward human hepatoma cell lines. Another study showed a leaf extract was cytotoxic toward T47D. Another study noted that the extracts have strong antiproliferation potential and can induce apoptosis. Another study showed pro-apoptosis of leaf extract on COLO-205. Another study showed mild cytotoxicity and inhibited cell proliferation of Capan-1. Another study showed the apoptotic effect of the acetogenin Annomuricin E on a form of colon cancer. Another study showed an extract decreased cell viability, inhibited cell proliferation, and induced cell death on MCF-7. A study showed the anti-proliferative and anticancer effects of crude extract on MCF-7, MDA-MB-231, and 4T1 cell lines. [343]

70

354. SOW THISTLE (Sonchus oleraceus)
Recommended Edible Plant: This lowly weed is actually edible, so toxicity is not a big concern. One study showed necrotic changes in cancer mass and possible activation of immune response on AM-3 cells. Another study showed growth inhibitory effects on all cancer cell lines tested.[344]

355. SPIDER FLOWER (Gynandropsis gynandra)
One study showed anticancer effect on hepatocellular carcinoma. Another study showed anticancer effects against EAC comparable to 5-FU. Another study isolated six cancer cell growth inhibitors including the known flavone Apigenin which inhibited P388 and all six compounds showed activity against all human cancer cell lines tested. Another study showed antiproliferative effects against lung and stomach cancer cell lines.[345]

356. SPREADING HOGWEED (Boerhavia diffusa) *IM
Recommended Edible Plant: Proper identification of the species is a must. One study showed the chemoprotective property of topical treatment of the extract on DMBA-induced skin papillomagenesis. Another study showed compounds in B. diffusa have anticancer potential to effectively inhibit the action of Bcl-2. Another study showed efficacy of a leaf extract against DAL in vivo. Another study showed cytotoxicity up to 96.3% against human papilloma virus type 16 infected SiHa cell line, the most common form of cervical cancer today. A study showed antiproliferative effects of a root extract on HeLa cells.[346]

357. ST. PAUL'S WORT (Siegesbeckia orientalis)
One study showed remarkable in vitro inhibition of the growth of HeLa cancer cells.[347]

358. STAR APPLE (Chrysophyllum cainito)
Top Recommended Edible Fruit: Not to be confused with the Star Fruit (Averrhoa carambola, also in this list) Star Apple is a small purple sphere but when cut in half at the equator a star shaped region holding the seeds is clearly visible in the cross-section. Most folks don't like the irritating sticky milky sap in the skin of the fruit which makes dealing with them a bit difficult, but Star Apple is one of the few fruits that has active phytochemicals that selectively target osteosarcoma (effective chemicals and plants against such Bone Cancers are RARE) and it is also a vasodilator and strengthens the blood as well. A study showed a polyphenolic fraction from the fruits induced apoptotic cell death in the U-2 ATCC HTB-96 cell line.[348]

359. STAR FRUIT (Averrhoa carambola)
Top Recommended Edible Fruit: Most people only know Star Fruit from its occasional availability in grocery stores, which are picked too green and loaded with Oxalic Acid which is toxic. Carambola should only be eaten fully tree ripened and then only occasionally. They still have some oxalic acid even fully tree-ripened (which are much sweeter) and there are reports that

people with kidney problems and renal failure have DIED from eating it: IF YOU HAVE KIDNEY ISSUES AVOID STAR FRUIT. A study of leaf extract showed cytotoxic activity against MCF-7. A study showed tumor inhibition of fruit extract on EAC cells in vivo via apoptosis and antiangiogenic activity attributed to Catechin, Epicatechin and Ferulic Acid.[349]

360. STINKVINE (Paederia foetida)
Recommended Edible Plant: Its name is due to the high sulfur content and it is slightly bitter but perfectly edible – young leaves and shoots farthest from the roots are best because the plant will absorb heavy metals from the soil. A study showed an extract had anticancer activity against human nasopharyngeal epidermoid carcinoma.[350]

361. STRAWBERRY (Fragaria vesca)
Top Recommended Edible Fruit: Strawberries have countless species, hybrids and cultivars, but all Strawberries contain similar anthocyanidins that have both antioxidant and anticancer power. Try to find organic strawberries and confirm that pesticides and more importantly fungicides were not used on them while fruiting and by the way, the "seeds" stuck to them are actually the fruits and what we call "strawberries" are actually just swollen stems.[62]

362. SUMA ROOT (Pfaffia paniculata) *IM
Top Recommended Holistic Herb: Sometimes called "Brazilian Ginseng" but only to cash in on the ginseng craze because it is not at all related to any of the plants traditionally called "Ginseng," this plant does have some studies dating back to the 1970's showing that it is an immunostimulant and has anticancer activity.[351]

363. SUNBERRY (Physalis minima)
Top Recommended Edible Fruit: Most species of Physalis (there are a lot including Cape Gooseberry, Chinese Lantern, Inca Berry and a famous close relative to them, Ashwagandha) are easily confused with each other and are also edible and contain unique kinds of compounds called Withanolides, Withaphysalins, and Physalins, all of which have health promoting powers and some exhibit potent anticancer properties as well. Studies have shown the anticancer efficacy of Sunberry on lung adenocarcinoma, colorectal carcinoma, Hep2, T47D, NSCLC, and HeLa.[352]

364. SWEET ACACIA (Acacia farnesiana)
Recommended Holistic Herb: There are hundreds of species of Acacia and closely related genera of trees. Their constituents vary greatly and substitutions (accidental or intentional) may be of inferior quality and effect. A study yielded four new diterpenoids including: Acasiane B, Farnesirane A, Farnesirane B and some were cytotoxic toward human cancer cell lines.[353]

365. SWEET BROOM (Scoparia dulcis) *IM
One study isolated Scopadulcic acid B, a diterpenoid that inhibited phospholipid synthesis and suppressed promotion of skin tumors induced by TPA. [354]

366. SWEET VIOLET (Viola odorata)
Two studies have shown anticancer efficacy but caution is advised since there was no discussion concerning general toxicity.[355]

367. TAILED MAIDENHAIR (Adiantum caudatum)
Recommended Edible Plant: Although the true Maidenhair fern (Adiantum capillus) is much more well known for its edibility in its native range, young fronds can be cooked like a vegetable. One study showed that extracts had high cytotoxicity against human gastric, colon, and breast cancer cell lines.[356]

368. TAIWAN GONIOTHALAMUS (Goniothalamus amuyon)
Almost all of the studies on this tree have been investigations into its anticancer properties and while the work is in the early stages, it looks like the plant does have future potential locked up in its unique phytochemicals. A study isolated Styrylpyrone Goniodiol-7-monoacetate, which showed potent cytotoxicity against KB, P-388, RPMI and TE671 tumor cells. A study of the leaves and stems yielded two new compounds: (6R,7R,8R)-8-methoxygoniodiol and (6R,7R,8R)-8-chlorogoniodiol, the second showed significant selective cytotoxicity toward HONE-1. Another study yielded three new compounds: Goniofupyrone A, Deoxygoniopypyrone A, and Digoniodiol, along with ten known compounds. Goniothalamin, Goniothalamin epoxide, and 8-Chlorogoniodiol showed cytotoxicity against the HepG2, Hep3B, MDA-MB-231, and MCF-7 cell lines. Goniothalamin has shown cytotoxicity against a wide range of cancers: breast, blood, ovary, lung, kidney, prostate, liver and colon. A study isolated Goniothalamin and showed it induced apoptosis in hepatocellular carcinoma. Another study showed the anticancer activities of Goniothalamin against NSCLC. Another study demonstrated how Goniothalamin triggers apoptosis in cancer cells.[357]

369. TAMARIND (Tamarindus indica)
Top Recommended Edible Fruit: Tamarind creates an ugly brown seed pod filled with large very hard shiny black seeds surrounded by a brown paste. It is that brown paste ranging from very sour to sweet-and-sour that is edible. It might be a bit of a fuss to eat, but it has shown potent neuroprotective power and the ability to neutralize fluoride (a well known NEUROTOXIN and a VERY RARE ability) making it well worth the effort. Leaf extracts have also been shown in preliminary laboratory studies to have promising anticancer effects as well.[358]

370. TANGLE FERN (Dicranopteris linearis)
Another edible fern, but expert identification of the species is a must. One study showed promising cytotoxic activity against HL-60 cell lines and it was found to be non-toxic to normal WRL 68 liver cells. [359]

371. TARO (Colocasia esculenta) *IM
Taro contains raphides which form microscopic crystals that produce irritation. Processed products should have been boiled

which neutralizes the raphides making these products safe. One study showed Taro may have a novel tumor specific anticancer activity. Another study showed antioxidant and anticancer activities against MCF-7.[360]

372. TEA (Camellia sinensis)
Top Recommended Holistic Herb: Tea contains a compound called EGCG which is an antioxidant about 100 TIMES stronger than Vitamin C and it has been shown in many studies to be one of the most effective anticancer compounds having antiangiogenic and antimetastatic properties, BUT overindulgence will literally RUIN any benefits it might bring. Tea is loaded with caffeine and tannins which have been shown to have detrimental effects in excess. One cup of hot tea per day is a maximum and I have known folks who pounded it down both hot and cold all day long and it led to kidney problems. You have been warned. Green tea is much higher in the Catechins and much lower in Tannins.[361]

373. THREE-LEAF CAYRATIA (Cayratia trifolia)
Recommended Edible Plant: This vine is eaten like a vegetable in India. One study isolated Epifriedelanol which showed antitumor activity. A study found 20 compounds of them Cyclopentadecane; 9-Borabicyclo [3.3.1] nonane; Oxirane; 9-(2-propen-1-yloxy)-1,4,8,12,16-Tetramethyl-heptadecan-4-olide; and Vitamin E may act as agonists for PPARγ as potential anticancer treatments. Another study found that Linoleic Acid, isolated from an extract, may act as a novel inhibitor of CXCR4, promising potential as a therapeutic for many types of cancer.[362]

374. THREE-LEAVED CHASTE TREE (Vitex trifolia)
All species of Vitex are potentially powerful holistic plants. This one contains a compound called Vitexicarpin which in two independent studies has shown promise against K562. Another study showed efficacy against both HepG2 and HeLa. Another study showed strong selective inhibition against MCF-7 and weak inhibition against the normal Vero cell line. [363]

375. THRYALLIS (Galphimia glauca)
A study of extracts yielded Galphimine B which selectively inhibits discharges of dopaminergic neurons in vivo. This study caused no deaths in the mice, no histopathic changes and all of the extracts inhibited colon cancer growth with no genotoxicity.[364]

376. TICKTREE (Desmodium gangeticum)
This plant has more studies than most in this list leading to a whole host of positive health benefits including its potential for use as an anticancer drug. Salicin, isolated from the plant, showed high binding affinity against COX-2 protein and lesser interaction with COX-1 and suggests it could be a potential COX inhibitor. Its anticancer activity was confirmed in vivo.[365]

377. TIGER'S CLAW (Erythrina variegata)
A study of a root bark extract in vivo showed a protective effect against DAL. Another study found a glycoside and 10,11-dioxo-

erythratidine in the leaves. The compounds showed anticancer activity in vitro against T47D. Another study isolated Xanthoxyletin which showed inhibitory effects on SGC-7901.[366]

378. TOMATO (Lycopersicon esculentum)
Top Recommended Edible Fruit: While studies have been inconclusive regarding its use to treat prostate cancer, there is no denying the tremendous health potential of Lycopene, a powerful tetraterpenoid antioxidant in the same family of compounds as beta-Carotene and it's what makes them red. With over 7,500 varieties most people want to know which ones are the best: "The redder; the better." So Beefsteak, Roma, and any other deep red varieties have the most Lycopene in them. Other studies have shown the power of Tomatoes to prevent DNA damage induced by well known chemical mutagens and also to prevent DNA damage from radiation. Load up on those tomatoes, they are not just good, they are good for you too. One study showed a broad spectrum of antimutagenic and anticlastogenic effects of the combination of tomato and garlic against DBMA-induced genetic damage and oxidative stress in vivo and highlighted the health benefits that can be achieved through combinations of functional (i.e. medicinal) foods. In another study, pretreatment with tomato extract resulted in a significant reduction in DNA damage caused by radiation exposure. Another study showed the antiproliferative activity of tomato leaf extract in vitro on C6.[10][65]

379. TORCH GINGER (Etlingera elatior)
Recommended Edible Plant: Flowers, flower buds and fruit are edible usually in soups and salads, though the fruit is said to be extremely sour and used in fish dishes. Studies have shown efficacy against B16, MCF-7, MDA-MB-231, and HT-29 cells.[367]

380. TOUCH-ME-NOT (Impatiens balsamina)
One study isolated, 2-methoxy-1,4-naphthoquinone, which showed intense anti-tumor activity against HepG2. Another study showed strong in vivo cytotoxicity against HeLa, and was found to be safe toward healthy cells indicating a very significant selective anti-tumor and cytotoxicity targeting only the cancerous cells. Another study isolated 2-methoxy-1,4-naphtho-quinone and showed the crude extract and isolated MeONQ exhibit protective effects on the pancreas, stomach, duodenum, and spleen in vivo indicating broad spectrum anticancer power. A study showed an extract was effective against HSC-2 via AMPK apoptosis.[368]

381. TREE BEAN (Parkia javanica)
Although the seed pods are edible there is no confirmation that they are completely nontoxic. Caution is advised. Two different studies confirmed anticancer effects against various cancer cell lines and one study showed apoptosis against S-180. [369]

382. TREE OF INDIA (Polyalthia longifolia) *IM
One study showed anticancer effects of fruit extracts against hepatocellular carcinoma in vivo.[370]

383. TREE OF LIFE (Platycladus orientalis)
This relative of pines, also called Arbor-vitae or Thuja, is a popular ornamental worldwide. It has been used for thousands of years by various cultures for sundry health benefits. One study confirmed its cytotoxicity on renal adenocarcinoma and amelanotic melanoma. A study showed anticancer potency against A549, SK-OV-3, A498 and HCT-15 cell lines. [371]

384. TRIDAX DAISY (Tridax procumbens)
Recommended Holistic Herb: One study showed potent anticancer activity of leaf extracts against A549 and HepG2.[372]

385. TROPICAL ALMOND (Terminalia catappa)
Top Recommended Edible Plant: Although not well known in the West, the nut is very popular in India. One study showed a leaf extract had significant anti-tumor effect against EAC. At least two studies have shown a significant antimetastatic property against liver carcinoma.[414]

386. TROPICAL CHICKWEED (Drymaria cordata)
Recommended Edible Plant: Another small weed that most folks would step over and never notice that is both edible and has enormous health benefits. It is nearly impossible to find for sale in any form like most common weeds, and expert identification is a must. A study showed cytotoxicity on HeLa and also isolated an anti-leukemic compound ($C_{17}H_{22}O_2$) effectively inhibitory toward human encomia cells.[373]

387. TURKEY-TAIL MUSHROOM (Trametes versicolor) *IM
Top Recommended Edible Mushroom: Like all of the gourmet edible mushrooms in this list, this one is also loaded with beta-Glucans which have been shown in numerous studies to have both immunostimulant and anticancer powers.[74][332]

388. TURMERIC (Curcuma longa)
Top Recommended Culinary Spice: Numerous studies have shown that Turmeric is antimutagenic and selectively targets and kills cancerous cells while providing support to healthy cells making Turmeric one of my Top Recommended Culinary herbs. Studies have shown it to be safe up to 2500mg/day in dietary supplements. Add Turmeric to soups, stews and casseroles and get a beautiful yellow color and add a wonderful earthy flavor to the food. A review of the biological activities lists in vitro anti-parasitic, anti-spasmodic, anti-inflammatory, gastroprotective and anticarcinogenesis and cancer growth inhibitory properties. A study of the oral administration of Curcumin and Curcumin plus Taxol significantly reduced breast cancer metastasis to the lung. A study showed cytotoxicity to lymphocytes and DAL. The active constituent was found to be Curcumin. Another study with human volunteers showed no hematological, renal or hepatic toxicity at 1 and 3 months. Turmeric extract has shown chemoprotective effect against chemically-induced malignancies in vivo. Another study showed that pretreatment with C. longa extract decreased all types

of chromosomal aberrations caused by radiation therapy. Another study of extracts showed potent growth suppressive activity on MCF-7. Another study in vivo showed anti-inflammatory, anti-proliferative and apoptotic effects against colon cancer.[374]

389. TURPETH TREE (Operculina turpethum)
One study showed an extract had antioxidant activity and a protective role against chemically induced breast cancer.[375]

390. VANILLA (Vanilla planifolia)
Top Recommended Culinary Spice: While whole Vanilla bean pods are sometimes available, the natural extract is the way to go. Studies have shown that Vanillin and Vanillic Acid have anticancer properties and the natural extract contains over 100 compounds many of which may have additional health benefits or a synergistic effect. Artificial Vanilla extract is pure Vanillin made by a synthetic process and may be effective, but the vast array of compounds in the natural products are always preferable.[376]

391. VELVET BEAN (Mucuna pruriens)
TOXIC: Well known for its L-dopa used in Parkinson's disease, Mucuna products must be properly processed to remove toxins. One study showed a decrease in tumor volume and viable cell count against EAC in vivo. [416]

392. VELVET LEAF (Cissampelos pareira) *IM
This is a climbing vine with clusters of beautiful red berries that are the only part of the plant to AVOID. Studies have shown the leaf extracts to be neuroprotective, hepatoprotective and also have potential in fighting cancers like KB and DAL.[377]

393. VERVAIN (Verbena officinalis)
Top Recommended Edible Plant: Leaves are cooked like a vegetable and used to make tea substitute. At least two studies have shown efficacy against cancer. Because the plant can be found in many well stocked garden centers and the work by many nurseries to hybridize the plant and create custom cultivars, expert identification of these plants is required.[378]

394. WAMPEE (Clausena lansium)
Top Recommended Edible Fruit: This close relative to the Pink Wampee (C. excavata, also in this list) has at least one study showing efficacy of the fruit as an anticancer agent and several others indicating potential anticancer properties in the leaves and stems. Clausenas look like grapes but are actually closely related to citrus which is evident when cut open revealing that they are segmented like citrus fruits.[379]

395. WANDERING ZEBRINA (Tradescantia zebrina)
Recommended Holistic Herb: This plant has some preliminary studies indicating it may have potent anticancer properties.[380]

396. WATER CRESS (Enhydra fluctuans)
Recommended Edible Plant: This is not the same species as the better known Net Negative Calorie food with the same name which is Nasturtium officinale. This is a floating aquatic plant and expert

identification of the species is a must. One study yielded two flavonoids: Baicalein 7-O-glucoside and Baicalein 7-O-diglucoside which showed significant anti-tumor activity against EAC.[381]

397. WATER HYACINTH (Eichhornia crassipes)
Recommended Edible Plant: A free-floating aquatic herb with long trailing roots, the surface leaves, and flowers are cooked and eaten like a vegetable. Several studies show some anticancer properties, but expert identification is necessary and stay away from the roots, the plant is considered very effective at removing heavy metals from contaminated waterways especially Lead and Cadmium both of which are highly toxic.[382]

398. WATER HYSSOP (Bacopa monnieri)
Top Recommended Holistic Herb: There are plenty of products and most call it "Bacopa." As with all "fad" plants verify that the product is not a substitution of another species. A study showed Bacopa monnieri has anticancer chemoprotective property against DBMA-induced skin papillomagenesis in vivo. [383]

399. WATER PENNYWORT (Hydrocotyle sibthorpioides)
Recommended Edible Plant: Water pennywort has a mildly mint-like flavor and can be used fresh like a condiment in soups, stews, and especially fish dishes. It has many studies showing that it promotes liver health. One study showed anti-tumor activity against S-180, and uterine cervical carcinoma comparable to the standard drug 5-FU. The extract also had immunomodulatory effects.[384]

400. WATER PLANTAIN (Ottelia alismoides)
Recommended Edible Plant: Most floating aquatic plants look the same to the untrained eye so expert verification of the species is a must. One study isolated Ottelione A and found it to be among the most potent natural compounds showing powerful antiproliferative activity against MCF-7, NCI-H460, and COLO205. [385]

401. WATER SPINACH (Ipomoea aquatica)
Although this vine, always found around ponds and slow-moving streams is edible, "Swamp cabbage" it is also a laxative. A study isolated the bioactive compound: 7-O-B-D-glucopyranosyl-dihydroquercetin-3-O-a-D-glucopyranoside (DHQG) which showed cytotoxicity towards all cancer cell lines tested.[386]

402. WHITE BERRY BUSH (Flueggea virosa)
Recommended Holistic/Edible Fruit: White Berry is not common so be sure to verify the species. One study yielded Fleuggine A and B. Fleuggine B showed growth inhibitory activity against MCF-7 and MDA-MB-231 cells. Another study showed high cytotoxicity and antiproliferative activity of Betulinic acid against the drug resistant K562/Adr cell line. [387]

403. WHITE FLOWERED MANGROVE (Lumnitzera racemosa)
Most species of mangrove (waterside trees with aerial roots) are TOXIC and I found no confirmation of this particular plant's toxicity. Two studies showed anticancer effects on HepG2 and HL-60.[388]

404. WILD HOPS (Flemingia strobilifera)
Can beer help fight cancer? Even if it could, ethanol is a terrible liver toxin nullifying any benefit it might bring. Best to try limited amounts of this plant in herbal teas and by the way this is a different species from the Hops used in flavoring beer which is also a potent herb. A study showed efficacy against MT-4.[389]

405. WILD RASPBERRY (Rubus moluccanus)
Top Recommended Edible Fruit: While I highly recommend this fruit, it is not related to raspberry which is a member of the Morus genus. This one is much harder to find for sale fresh, but it is worth the effort to find it or grow your own. Some extracts of Rubus spp. have shown moderate COX inhibitory activity and great potential to inhibit cancer cell growth (colon, breast, lung, and gastric human tumor cell lines) due to the high anthocyanidin content of the fruits. Another study of the fruit yielded eight 19-a-hydroxyursane-type compounds. Hyptatic Acid and 4-epi-Nigaichigoside F1 exhibited growth inhibition against colon tumor cells.[390]

406. WILD TEA (Ehretia microphilla)
Recommended Edible Plant: Not to be confused with commercial green and black tea (Camelia sinensis) this herb's leaves are often used as a substitute and it is commercially available. An added bonus if you can grow your own is that the fruits are edible. The tea has shown evidence that it has anticancer properties.[391]

407. WINGED TREEBINE (Cissus quadrangularis)
Recommended Holistic Herb: This plant is in a lot of weight-loss herbal products on the market and while it is certainly effective in this usage it also has been shown in studies to induce apoptosis in the HeLa cell line.[392]

408. WINTER ASTER (Chrysanthemum indicum)
Top Recommended Medicinal/Edible Herb: Exceedingly few such flowering ornamentals turn out to be completely safe in large doses for extended periods of time; this is one of them and it has a whole slew of health benefits as well as anticancer properties. And overindulgence is still not recommended despite studies showing it to be safe. A study showed significant selective apoptotic effect in MHCC97H cells without effecting normal cells. A study showed anti-metastatic effect on hepatocellular carcinoma. Two additional studies showed inhibition of proliferation and significant apoptotic effect on human hepatocellular carcinoma cells. In another study a flower extract prevented free radical-induced DNA damage and showed no toxicity. Another study reported the antiproliferative effect of the flower extract on A549. A study demonstrated the effect on signaling pathways as a possible source of its apoptotic power on different tumor cell lines. Be careful of substitutions and hybrids in all common flowering ornamentals like this one.[393]

409. WIRE GRASS (Eleusine indica)
A study of extracts of E. indica showed selective growth inhibition against human lung cancer and HeLa cell lines.[394]

410. WIREBUSH (Melochia corchorifolia)
Recommended Holistic/Edible Plant: A study of the extract of edible parts showed significant antioxidant and antiproliferative properties versus MCF7 cancer cells.[395]
411. WORMWOOD (Artemisia vulgaris)
Artemisia has a long and sordid history of abuse in Europe for its narcotic effects, but as long as you don't overindulge and in fact keep your exposure limited, it can have positive health benefits. One study showed aqueous extracts inhibited cell growth and colony formation of prostate, breast, and colorectal cancer cells. Another study of the oil showed apoptosis in HL-60 cell lines. Another study showed anticancer activity against HCT-15.[396]
412. YARD-LONG BEAN (Vigna unguiculata)
Top Recommended Edible Plant: Family to the ubiquitous green bean which may share some of the phytochemical constituents; these bean pods are up to 3 feet long. The antifungal peptide, Sesquin, showed antiproliferative activity on MCF-7 and M1.[397]
413. YARROW (Achillea millefolium)
Top Recommended Holistic Herb: Well known since ancient times, this plant has been a main stay in the holistic herbal medicine cabinet. Modern studies report some potential medicinal properties and at least two show possible anticancer potential against P-388 as well as antimutagenic power. Overindulgence can lead to health issues. CAUTION IS ADVISED.[398]
414. YELLOW-EYED GRASS (Sisyrinchium palmifolium)
Recommended Edible Plant: Rhizomes are collected dried and powdered and made into herbal teas that are considered both delicious as well as medicinal. Proper identification of the plant and verification of herbal products is a must. One study isolated 15 compounds, including 4 new glucosides, Eleutherinosides B to E. Two compounds showed inhibition of SW480 cells and selective cytotoxicity against three colorectal cancer cell lines.[399]
415. YELLOW SANCHEZIA (Sanchezia speciosa)
One study showed anticancer efficacy against MCF-7 and SK-MEL-5. Another study showed efficacy against HeLa.[400]
416. YERBA BUENA (Mentha arvensis)
Top Recommended Culinary Spice: Although well known in certain regions as a fresh leaf spice added to salads as well as used in cooking, in the U.S. it is more often used as a holistic medicinal herb. Nevertheless it is quite suitable for either use and it has at least one study showing that it might have anticancer properties as well.[401]
417. YLANG-YLANG (Cananga odorata)
This tree produces some of the most beautiful if not weird looking flowers. They are yellow with long drooping fleshy twisted petals that look like twisted yellow banana peels. The plant is the source of Cananga Oil used in aromatherapy and perfumes. A new sesquiterpene alkaloid, Cananodine, and two new sesquiterpenes

were isolated from the fruits of Ylang-ylang and were evaluated for cytotoxicity against two human hepatocarcinoma cell lines.[402]

418. ZEDOARY (Curcuma zedoaria)

Top Recommended Culinary Spice: Not nearly as common or well known as its intensely yellow relative Turmeric, Zedoary shares a lot of significant active phytochemistry with it including the "Curcuminoids" which are under investigation for both their antimutagenic and anticancer activity. Zedoary is considered relatively safe although a few cases of poisoning have been reported likely due to extreme overindulgence (eating it as a main dietary staple, rather than using it as a spice.) Five independent studies have shown anticancer power against murine melanoma, OVCAR-3, DAL, NSCLC, and SGC-7901 cell lines.[403]

THE IMMUNOSTIMULANTS

Several plants in the above list have immunostimulant activity as well as anticancer properties and a couple of them may get their anticancer power from the fact that they have a powerful effect on the immune system. As such, any immunostimulant holistic herb could turn out to be beneficial in cancer prevention and even have direct cancer fighting potential. Even if they don't have any direct anticancer power, they are still an excellent line up to help those folks who are undergoing the rigors of chemotherapy which wrecks the immune system and these plants can definitely help those patients recover much faster and help prevent them from getting other infections that can severely complicate their condition. These plants are either well respected as known immune boosters in the holistic medicinal circles or have at least one study proving the immunostimulant property. The ***AC** notation indicates the plant is also in the preceding Anticancer Plants List.

1. ACAI BERRY (Euterpe oleracea)

Top Recommended Edible Fruit: Acai is loaded with antioxidants and is an immunostimulant. Açai has become a "fad" plant and products are mixed with other fruits; find 100% pure products.[404]

2. AGARICUS BLAZEI MUSHROOM *AC

Top Recommended Edible Mushroom: All Edible Mushrooms are at the top of this list because of their beta-Glucans. Studies have proven that these are powerful immunostimulants and cancer fighters too. Each species has a different mixture of beta-Glucans in them which can have a significant impact on their benefits and potency. I highly recommend a related species; Agaricus bisporus, Button Mushrooms and Portabella Mushrooms (the same species) and all of the gourmet mushrooms in these two lists. [22][74][332]

3. ALFALFA (Medicago sativa) *AC

Alfalfa is a well known health and vigor tonic and studies have shown that it interferes with immunosuppressants indicating that it has strong immunostimulatory power. DO NOT USE ALFALFA IF YOU ARE TAKING IMMUNOSUPPRESSANTS. Overindulgence is NOT RECOMMENDED.[19]

4. ALOE (Aloe vera) *AC

Top Recommended Holistic Herb: Aside from studies showing Aloe-emodin to have measurable anticancer effects, another study isolated a new polysaccharide called Aloeride which has marked immunostimulant activity as well. Overindulgence of Aloe is NOT RECOMMENDED, it can over time cause liver damage. Take it in small doses every other day (500mg) or larger doses less often (i.e. one cup of pure juice every one to three weeks.)[33]

5. ARROWROOT (Maranta arundinacea)

A starchy root that is a staple food source in many countries, extracts showed significant immunostimulant effects.[405]

6. ANDROGRAPHIS (Andrographis paniculata) *AC

Top Recommended Holistic Herb: Despite being a fad plant, Andrographis has been shown to be an immunostimulant.[36]

7. ASTRAGALUS (Astragalus membranaceus) *AC

Top Recommended Holistic Herb: Yet another fad plant of late that is also an immunostimulant.[55]

8. BARLEY GRASS (Hordeum vulgare)

Top Recommended Superfood: Young Barley grass shoots are one of the most nutrient dense foods on Earth. One tablespoon contains high amounts of: Vitamin A (as beta-carotene,) Vitamin B1, B2, B3, B7, Copper, Iron, and Magnesium. It also provides significant amounts of: Betaine, Boron, Lutein, Alpha-Linoleic Acid (ALA, the plant Omega-3,) Oryzanol, Potassium, Selenium, Zinc, and various tocopherol forms of Vitamin E. It is a very rich source of Chlorophyll which triggers liver detoxification and it helps to reduce bad cholesterol, lowers blood pressure, boosts the immune system and many health professionals believe that a chlorophyll-rich diet may significantly reduce your risk of cancer.[14][64]

9. BEACH MORNING GLORY (Ipomoea pes-caprae)

Expert Identification of the species is required: Many species of Morning Glory vine (genus: Ipomoea) are TOXIC. One study demonstrated that I. pes-caprae caused significant proliferation of human T-lymphocytes in vivo.[406]

10. BISHOP'S WEED (Trachyspermum ammi)

Top Recommended Holistic Herb: Bishops weed, a.k.a. Ajwain, is related to some common spices and is used as such so it is relatively safe and it has been shown to have immunostimulatory properties.[419]

11. BLACK MYROBALAN (Terminalia chebula) *AC

Top Recommended Edible Plant: Featured in the Ayurvedic tradition of India. It has been shown in studies to be a strong immunostimulant.[78]

12. BONESET (Eupatorium perfoliatum) *AC

Top Recommended Holistic Herb: Boneset was very popular a hundred years ago for good reason. It is a strong immunostimulant as well as analgesic given by doctors for the pain of "Bone-break fever" (Dengue) hence the name.)[79]

13. BORAGE (Borago officinalis) *AC
Top Recommended Holistic Herb: Borage Oil has one of the highest concentrations of gamma-Linoleic Acid (an Omega-6 Fatty Acid) that has been shown to have both immunostimulant and anticancer properties.[80]

14. BUPLEURUM (Bupleurum chinense)
This herb has a history of use in Traditional Chinese Medicine and it is a strong immunostimulant.[420]

15. BUTTON MUSHROOM (Agaricus bisporus) *AC
Top Recommended Edible Mushroom: Even though all of the other gourmet mushrooms have more beta-Glucans in them, plain white Button Mushrooms found in any well stocked grocery store's produce section are no slouches: they average over 6300mg per cup (almost 7.5% by weight,) so this is no "trace ingredient;" they are loaded with them. Beta-Glucans have been shown in plenty of studies to be powerful immunostimulants and also actively combat certain forms of cancer.[30][74][332]

16. CAPERS (Capparis zeylanica)
Top Recommended Edible Plant: At least one study showed significant immunostimulatory activity and capers have the highest concentrations of the antioxidant flavonoids Quercetin and Kaempferol of any readily available edible plant (both proven cancer fighters) making capers a good addition to your dietary regimen.[421]

17. CAT'S CLAW (Uncaria tomentosa)
Top Recommended Holistic Herb: A huge vine found in the Amazonia Region where it is called "Uña de Gato," alkaloids in the plant have been shown to increase immune response by as much as 50% which has made it a prescription treatment by doctors in South America for immune deficiency diseases such as HIV and those undergoing chemotherapy for the treatment of cancer. [422]

18. CATUABA (Erythroxylum catuaba)
At least one study has shown this herb to have immunostimulatory properties. It is a close relative to the Coca plant, by the way.[423]

19. CELANDINE (Chelidonium majus) *AC
At least one study has shown this herb has immunostimulatory properties.[103]

20. CHAGA MUSHROOM (Inonotus obliquus) *AC
This is one of the expensive gourmet mushrooms that actually is difficult to grow because it is a parasite to certain species of trees and eventually kills them, but it is potent medicine and loaded with those valuable beta-Glucans that have been shown to be powerful immunostimulants and cancer fighters. Beware of products that are fractions (partial extracts) and find 100% pure dried powder instead.[74][106][332]

21. CHAMOMILE (Matricaria recutita)
Top Recommended Holistic Herb: At least one study showed that Chamomile stimulates the immune system so it can ward off

infection while not introducing any effects that could aggravate the condition. Chamomile is considered very safe and is usually made into herbal teas.[424]

22. CHANCA PIEDRA (Phyllanthus niruri) *AC

Top Recommended Holistic Herb: Although it is a verified immunostimulant it is best known for its power to break up kidney and urinary tract stones. Science is currently studying the active compounds for possible use in treatment of Hepatitis and HIV so it does have strong antiviral potential likely due to immune system activity. It is powerful medicine: USE IN MODERATION.[108]

23. CHICORY (Cichorium intybus) *AC

Top Recommended Edible Plant: Often used as a coffee substitute and well known for its ability to detoxify the system of Uric acid (causes Gout) and to help the liver, it contains Inulin which has been shown to act as an immunostimulant. While relatively safe, it should be used in moderation because it is powerful medicine. Do not use it if you have or have ever had trouble with gall stones.[113]

24. CHINESE BELL FLOWER (Abutilon indicum) *AC

This plant has numerous studies showing a wide range of health benefits including significant immunostimulatory effects.[115]

25. COCONUT (Cocos nucifera) *AC

Top Recommended Edible Plant: Coconut is well known for its many health benefits and contains Capric, Lauric and Caprylic Acids (RARE Nutritional Fatty Acids) in abundance that have been shown to promote various health benefits and it is considered an immunostimulant. You can drink the water, milk, or eat the solid white meat. The oil is a good substitute for any other oil in cooking because it is stable at high temperatures.[37]

26. COLEUS (Plectranthus barbatus) *AC

Top Recommended Holistic Herb: Coleus contains Forskolin which is well studied and a proven powerful immunostimulant and is already prescribed to cancer patients undergoing chemotherapy. Forskolin has a very powerful effect on lowering blood pressure and must not be taken by anyone on blood pressure, blood thinner or cholesterol medications. Forskolin also induces stomach acid secretion and should not be used by anyone suffering from gastric problems. Obviously Coleus extract supplements should be used in moderation.[132]

27. COMMON COCKSCOMB (Celosia argentea) *AC

Already in the Anticancer plant list and this plant has also been proven to have immunostimulatory effects.[133]

28. COMMON LEUCAS (Leucas aspera) *AC

Another plant in the anticancer plant list that has at least one study demonstrating strong immunostimulant activity.[134]

29. COPTIS (Coptis sinensis) *AC

The Chinese species is far more common than the one found in North America which is actually an endangered species. Coptis is a well known COX Inhibitor making it a strong anti-inflammatory and it is also suspected of being a very strong immunostimulant because of this effect. Small doses increase alertness, brain function and blood pressure. Larger doses induce drowsiness and lower blood pressure. You should consult a professional herbalist to determine the right dosage to use.[136]

30. CORIANDER (Coriandrum sativum) *AC
Top Recommended Culinary Spice: Used for thousands of years in India in the traditional Ayurvedic medicinal practices, Coriander is a well known immune system booster. Coriander is the ground seed of the same plant whose leaves are sold as Cilantro. The ground seed is a bit bitter, but it is far stronger than Cilantro for its immunostimulant effects. Coriander is completely safe and an excellent spice to use in soups, stews, etc.[127]

31. CUT-LEAVED PANAX (Polyscias fruticosa)
Rarely seen outside of its native ranges, this plant is used like Celery and Parsley and it has at least one study confirming its immunostimulatory properties. [425]

32. DANG SHEN (Codonopsis pilosula)
Top Recommended Holistic Herb: Codonopsis has a long history of use in Traditional Chinese Medicine and it is an immunostimulant and also a vasodilator which helps to lower blood pressure. Those taking blood pressure medication should not use it. Other than that it is considered relatively safe.[426]

33. DATES (Phoenix dactylifera)
Top Recommended Edible Plant: At least one study showed immunostimulant effects.[427]

34. DONG QUAI (Angelica sinensis)
Top Recommended Holistic Herb: Chinese Angelica is loaded with phytoestrogens and is well known for treating women's health issues, but it has been shown to stimulate the production of white blood cells making it a potent immunostimulant. Dong Quai also has confirmed blood purifying, anti-inflammatory and liver protective powers. Although relatively safe, it should not be used by pregnant women or anyone suffering from any viral infection. Prolonged excessive use is not recommended.[152]

35. DURIAN (Durio zibethinus)
Top Recommended Edible Plant: This fruit has gained some notoriety due to its terrible stench, but those who have tried it say it tastes exquisite. Rind supplements are a better choice because they contain an unusual polysaccharide that has been shown to have immunostimulant power.[428]

36. DWARF GEOMETRY TREE (Bucida spinosa)
This plant's main usage in holism is for its immunostimulant effects which have been demonstrated in at least one study.[429]

37. ECHINACEA (Echinacea angustifolia)
Top Recommended Edible Plant: E. purpurea and E. pallida are also used. Studies have shown that there are many phytonutrients

in the plant that play a synergistic role in boosting the immune system. Most experts agree that it is most effective in prevention or in the earliest stages of cold and flu and once the illness is in full swing it does not appear to be very effective. But, Echinacea does have immunostimulant properties and is considered relatively safe. If you have an autoimmune disease such as rheumatoid arthritis or Lupus, or if you suffer from a chronic infection like Tuberculosis or HIV or if you are allergic to ragweed (it is a close relative) then you must not use Echinacea.[430]

38. ELEUTHERO (Eleutherococcus senticosus)
Top Recommended Holistic Herb: A.k.a. Siberian Ginseng, Eleuthero has a long tradition of use in Chinese medicine as a health tonic and it is a strong immunostimulant. It is also well known for increasing brain function, concentration and alertness without the negative side effects of stimulants like caffeine. It is relatively safe with lower negative side effects than Asian or American Ginseng and it is also a good adaptogen which helps the body deal with sudden dramatic changes such as those going on a calorie restricted diet and comes highly recommended. Moderation is advised. Not for long-term use. [431]

39. ELECTRIC DAISY (Spilanthes acmella)
A study of this unusual landscaping flower has demonstrated its immunostimulatory effects.[432]

40. ENOKI MUSHROOM (Flammulina veluptis) *AC
Top Recommended Holistic/Edible Mushroom: All of the gourmet mushrooms are loaded with the beta-Glucans, powerful immunostimulants and cancer fighters. Only buy 100% pure dried powders.[74][332]

41. EPIMEDIUM (Epimedium grandiflorum)
Horny Goat Weed has a long history of use in Traditional Chinese Medicine as an aphrodisiac and treatment for male impotence, but it is also a strong immunostimulant. MODERATION IS HIGHLY RECOMMENDED: in excess it can increase blood pressure and heart rate.[433]

42. EVENING PRIMROSE (Oenothera biennis)
Top Recommended Holistic Herb: The roots are edible and the plant has good nutritional value and has anti-inflammatory and immunomodulatory power due mainly to the presence of Gamma-Linoleic Acid. Excessive use of the Seed Oil (the most commonly available product) can cause bloating and digestive upset so moderation is advised.[434]

43. FALSE PRIMROSE (Ludwigia octovalvis) *AC
One study showed non-toxicity and significant immunostimulatory effects.[168]

44. FEVER BARK (Alstonia scholaris) *AC
Also in the Anticancer plants list, Fever Bark has been shown to be a strong immunostimulant. MODERATION IS ADVISED: not for long-term continual use.[170]

45. FO-TI (Polygonum multiflorum)
Top Recommended Holistic Herb: Fo-ti root has powerful immunomodulatory and immunostimulatory effects that are of great interest to those suffering from cancer and going through chemotherapy. MODERATION IS ADVISED.[177]

46. GALANGAL GINGER (Alpinia galanga) *AC
Top Recommended Holistic Herb: Another powerful plant from the Anticancer plant list that has been shown in at least one study to have immunostimulant effects.[185]

47. GHOST FLOWER (Aeginetia indica) *AC
One study showed that this unusual parasitic flower does have immunostimulatory properties.[188]

48. GINGER (Zingiber officinale) *AC
Top Recommended Culinary Spice: Don't be fooled by the seemingly exaggerated reputation, Ginger has been shown to have immunostimulant properties along with an impressive list of healing powers most of which have been verified in scientific studies.[190]

49. GINKGO BILOBA
Top Recommended Holistic Herb: This Traditional Chinese Medicinal herb has numerous scientific studies showing that it does increase circulation and enhances the efficiency of the "Blood-brain barrier" allowing more oxygen to reach the brain cells enhancing brain function. It is also believed to be a longevity tonic and a powerful immune booster. If you are on blood thinners, blood pressure, cholesterol medication or MAO Inhibitor drugs you must not take Ginkgo.[435]

50. GINSENG (Panax ginseng)
This is probably one of the least understood holistic herbs. It is a powerful restorative tonic and a potent immunostimulant ideal for those who are convalescing due to chronic illness, fatigue, or debilitation. Do not use Ginseng if you suffer from high blood pressure or are on blood pressure, blood thinner, or cholesterol medication. Moderation is advised and continual use is not recommended because Ginseng is very strong medicine and should only be used to recuperate.[436]

51. GOJI BERRY (Lycium chinensis) *AC
Top Recommended Edible Plant: Most products are Wolfberry (L. barbatum) which is similar in appearance but the bushes have far better yields than true Goji berry bushes which is why the substitution is almost always made. Hold out for the real thing which is a powerful antioxidant and strong immunostimulant.[39]

52. GOLDEN EYE GRASS (Curculigo orchioides) *AC
Also in the Anticancer plant list, at least one study has confirmed the rhizomes have immunostimulant properties as well.[195]

53. GOLDENSEAL (Hydrastis canadensis)
Although edible, the leaves and roots are very bitter and it is best used as a digestive aid and long-term use is not recommended.

Goldenseal contains many unique compounds like Hydrastine but, it also contains Berberine and Chlorogenic acid, both of which have studies demonstrating potent anticancer properties and the plant is suspected of being an immunostimulant as well.[437]

54. GUAVA (Psidium guajava) *AC

Top Recommended Superfood: One fruit provides 100% RDA of Vitamin C and one study showed it does have immunostimulatory effects.[81]

55. HEAVENLY ELIXIR (Tinospora crispa)

Close relatives of T. crispa may also possess the demonstrated immunostimulant effects of this popular holistic herb. Cardiac patients should avoid using the Tinosporas.[438]

56. HOLY BASIL (Ocimum tenuiflorum) *AC

Top Recommended Holistic Herb: Holy Basil is already in the Anticancer List with promising results. One study showed that it increased antibody production and cellular immune response in vivo.[206]

57. HONEYBUSH (Cyclopia spp.) *AC

Top Recommended Holistic Herb: Also in the Anticancer list, Honeybush has been shown to be an effective immunostimulant and is one of the safest herbal teas available.[208]

58. HUMMINGBIRD BUSH (Hamelia patens) *AC

Also in the Anticancer plants list, one study showed that it also has significant immunostimulatory effects.[209]

59. INDIAN HELIOTROPE (Heliotropium indicum) *AC

An in vivo study showed increased lymphocyte viability and higher concentrations of antibodies.[407]

60. INDIGO (Indigofera tinctoria) *AC

Indigo has been shown to have immunostimulant properties.[216]

61. IXORA (Ixora coccinea) *AC

Aside from studies showing anticancer properties, one study confirmed the immunostimulant power of the flowers. Who knew Ixora has such amazing health potential?[222]

62. JIAOGULAN (Gynostemma pentaphyllum)

Top Recommended Holistic Herb: This is another Traditional Chinese Medicinal herb with a legendary reputation as a health and longevity tonic. It is a powerful immunostimulant, adaptogen, vasodilator and lowers blood pressure. If you are on high blood pressure medication do not take Jiaogulan. [439]

63. JOSHUA TREE (Yucca spp.) *AC

Top Recommended Holistic Herb: This desert plant's roots have saponins which have been shown in studies and even applied medicine manufacture to have immunostimulant properties. Desert or Mojave Yucca is best used in prepared product capsules with specific dosages because saponins can turn toxic in excess.[231]

64. JUDAS EAR (Auricularia auricula-judae) *AC

Top Recommended Edible Mushroom: The edible mushrooms are all under investigation for their enormous potential health benefits mainly due to their unique polysaccharides called beta-Glucans which have proven potent anticancer, tumor inhibitory and immunostimulant properties. [74][228]

65. JUJUBE (Ziziphus jujuba) *AC

Top Recommended Edible Plant: Although the study showing immunostimulant activity was done with a leaf extract the fruit is very healthy and when sun-dried, tastes like dates.[232]

66. LEMON (Citrus limonum) *AC

Top Recommended Edible Plant: Lemons (and Limes) are high in Vitamin C and other phytonutrients called Limonoids that may have significant anticancer and immune boosting power. Add lemon to other herbal teas to improve the taste and a glass of Lemonade once in a while is an excellent thirst quencher and powerful holistic medicine.[246]

67. LUFFA (Luffa cylindrica)

Top Recommended Edible Plant: This gourd is cooked like a vegetable and also sun-dried and made into sponges! One study demonstrated its immunostimulatory effects.[440]

68. MACA ROOT (Lepidium peruvianum)

Top Recommended Holistic Herb: Maca is an edible root tuber or rhizome of a tropical vine and is a staple food in some South American regions. In those regions it also has a reputation of being an energy tonic and there is evidence that it may be a good immunostimulant. It has high concentrations of phytoestrogens and can help with women's health issues. Like all such plants it could exacerbate existing hormone-dependent cancers.[441]

69. MAITAKE MUSHROOM (Grifola frondosa) *AC

Top Recommended Holistic/Edible Mushroom: This is another gourmet mushroom loaded with beta-Glucans that have been proven to be powerful immunostimulants and cancer fighters. Beware of fractions (partial extracts) and look for 100% pure dried powder instead.[74][254][332]

70. MANGO (Mangifera indica) *AC

Top Recommended Edible Plant: At least one study has shown it to have immunostimulant effects.[45]

71. NICKER TREE (Caesalpinia bonducella) *AC

Nicker Tree seeds have been shown to have immunostimulant effects.[270]

72. NONI (Morinda citrifolia) *AC

Top Recommended Holistic Herb: The key to Noni's health potential seems to be several unique phytonutrients including its oligosaccharides which are not the same as the beta-Glucans found in mushrooms, but like them, they are complex sugars and studies have shown that they could have similar immunostimulant and even anticancer powers. [273]

73. OATS (Avena sativa)

Top Recommended Edible Plant: On the subject of the beta-Glucans, Oatmeal is one of the only other sources of them other than edible mushrooms and there has already been plenty of scientific research proving that the beta-Glucans are powerful immunostimulants and anticancer compounds. Aside from being high in dietary fiber which helps the digestive tract and reduces the absorption of cholesterol, Oats also bring Manganese, some B vitamins, and are the only thing you should be eating for breakfast because they bring these valuable beta-Glucans as well.[15]

74. ORCHID TREE (Bauhinia variegata) *AC
Already in the Anticancer plants list, it has also been shown to have immunostimulant effects.[277]

75. OREGON GRAPE ROOT (Mahonia aquifolium)
Top Recommended Holistic Herb: This holistic herb is a source of Berberine which has already been shown in studies to have powerful anticancer properties and the plant is also a strong immunostimulant. Extracts are not quite as good as whole fresh root products which contain tannins that have an anti-inflammatory effect. Continual use is NOT RECOMMENDED and it should not be taken if you suffer from chronic gastrointestinal infections or other digestive problems like Irritable Bowel Syndrome.[442]

76. OYSTER MUSHROOM (Pleurotus spp.) *AC
Top Recommended Holistic/Edible Mushroom: By now you know the story: beta-Glucans, and all edible mushrooms are loaded with these powerful immunostimulants that also actively combat cancer. Only buy 100% pure dried powder. [74][332]

77. PAPAYA (Carica papaya) *AC
Top Recommended Edible Plant: Papaya has at least one study of the fruit showing that it has immunostimulatory effects.[47]

78. PAU D'ARCO (Tabebuia spp.) *AC
Top Recommended Holistic Herb: The inner bark of several species of Tabebuia is indeed powerful medicine and it is believed that regular usage by natives in the Amazonia region is what makes them immune to Malaria and other infectious diseases. There is not enough research into this plant to be sure, but it does look like it has potent immunostimulant and/or immunomodulatory powers. Moderation is advised.[284]

79. POMEGRANATE (Punica granatum) *AC
Top Recommended Edible Plant: Already in the Anticancer list because of many compounds that have proven anticancer powers including Punicic Acid, Palmitic Acid, Chlorogenic Acid, Linoleic Acid, Oleic Acid, and a group of unique phytonutrients called Punicalagins, Pomegranate is also an immunostimulant. Fresh squeezed is best, but commercially available juice products are loaded with antioxidants and these powerful phytonutrients too.[56]

80. PORCUPINE FLOWER (Barleria prionitis)
This plant has at least one study showing it has immunostimulant effects.[443]

81. PORTABELLA MUSHROOM (Agaricus bisporus) *AC
Top Recommended Edible Mushroom: See Button Mushroom.

82. PORTULACA (Portulaca grandiflora)
Top Recommended Edible Plant: Closely related to several other species in the Anticancer list and likely possessing similar properties, Portulaca, the very popular flower found in many well stocked garden centers has one study demonstrating its strong immunostimulant properties. Cook well; it has Calcium oxalate crystals in it which are toxic but neutralized by boiling.[444]

83. PRICKLY CHAFF FLOWER (Achyranthes aspera)
At least one study demonstrated this plant's immunostimulatory effects.[445]

84. PUMPKIN SEED (Cucurbita maxima)
Top Recommended Superfood: Pumpkin seeds are an excellent source of minerals like Zinc and have been shown in at least one study to have measurable immunostimulant effects.[11]

85. RED COTTON (Bombax ceiba) *AC
At least one study showed this plant's immunostimulatory effects and it is also in the Anticancer plants list. There is no mention of potential toxicity so moderation is advised.[307]

86. REISHI MUSHROOM (Ganoderma lucidum) *AC
Top Recommended Holistic Mushroom: Reishi mushrooms have one of the highest concentrations of beta-Glucans, powerful immunostimulants and cancer fighters, but look for 100% pure dried powder, never, fractions or mixtures which will be DILUTED with cheaper constituents.[74][311][332]

87. RHODIOLA (Rhodiola rosea)
Top Recommended Holistic Herb: Rhodiola is an adaptogen and as expected it is also a strong immunostimulant known in both Eastern and Western cultures for thousands of years. Use as directed or even smaller doses because it can become a strong sedative in larger doses. Do not use if you suffer from pathological mental disorders such as bipolar disorder.[409]

88. ROOIBOS (Aspalathus linearis) *AC
Top Recommended Holistic Herb: Rooibos is one of the safest herbal teas in this book and it is also a known immunostimulant. Despite being perfectly safe, moderation is recommended.[314]

89. ROSEMARY (Rosmarinus officinalis) *AC
Top Recommended Culinary/Holistic Herb: Rosemary contains Rosmarinic Acid and studies have shown it is immunomodulatory and an antidepressant.[317]

90. SARSAPARILLA (Smilax sarsaparilla) *AC
Sarsaparilla root is anti-inflammatory, effective against arthritis and gout by neutralizing endotoxins found in the blood of people with these afflictions and it may well help bolster the immune system. Chronic usage is not recommended. Moderation is advised.[123]

91. SCARLET BUSH (Hamelia patens)
This plant contains Rosmarinic Acid which has been shown to have both an immunomodulatory and antidepressant effect (See Rosemary.) It also contains Pteropodine and Isopeteropodine, two

alkaloids found to have immunostimulant properties.[408]

92. SCHISANDRA (Schisandra chinensis)

Top Recommended Edible Plant: Schisandra berries have a long legendary history in Traditional Chinese Medicine and are loaded with antioxidants and other unique phytonutrients and are a powerful immunostimulant. Specialty Chinese Grocery stores might carry them, but it is a fast growing vine and you could grow your own. Overindulgence is not recommended as they could cause upset stomach and they may contain phytoestrogens.[446]

93. SEA BUCKTHORN (Hippophae rhamnoides)

Top Recommended Edible Plant: The main constituents are impressive: Vitamin C, Beta-Carotene, Beta-Sitosterol, Lycopene, Isorhamnetin, Kaempferol, Linoleic Acid, Malic Acid, Oleic Acid, and Quercetin. Many of those compounds have been shown in studies to have anticancer properties and it is loaded with many well known antioxidants like beta-Carotene and Lycopene and it is also an immunostimulant. It is definitely on the menu though you will likely only find the Fruit Oil which is very good and can be taken internally and has a reputation of being not only safe but very healthy too.[447]

94. SEA ROSEMALLOW (Hibiscus tiliaceus) *AC

One study showed this Hibiscus species has immunostimulant effects. [326]

95. SHIITAKE MUSHROOMS (Lentinus edodes) *AC

Top Recommended Holistic/Edible Mushroom: Chaga, Maitake Shiitake, and Reishi have the highest concentrations of beta-Glucans, powerful immunostimulants and cancer fighters but look for 100% pure dried powder, not fractions or mixtures which will be DILUTED with cheaper ingredients.[74][332]

96. SPEARGRASS (Imperata cylindrica)

This is another plant with unusual polysaccharides similar to the beta-Glucans that have shown immunostimulant effects.[448]

97. SPIRULINA (Arthrospira platensis)

Top Recommended Superfood: Spirulina, or Blue Green Algae, has a very strong taste, but dried spirulina is a superfood and 3 to 4 oz, per day will fulfill 100% RDA requirements of Iron and several essential Vitamins. It is also a potent immunostimulant and it is perfectly safe, but brings too much Copper which can become toxic in excess.[13]

98. SPREADING HOGWEED (Boerhavia diffusa) *AC

At least one study verified its immunostimulatory effects.[346]

99. SUGAR CANE (Saccharum offinarum)

Top Recommended Edible Plant: The Cuban community makes a drink called "Guarapo" which is just squeezed raw sugar cane. This has been shown to have immunostimulant effects and is a healthy refreshing sweet drink unlike processed white sugar which is a known cause of Type II Diabetes and has also been shown to increase the risk of cancer. [449]

100. SUMA ROOT (Pfaffia paniculata) *AC
Top Recommended Holistic Herb: Already in the Anticancer plant list, this holistic herb is also a potent immunostimulant. While it is edible and has no reports of toxicity, it is a stimulant and moderation is advised.[351]

101. SWEET BROOM (Scoparia dulcis) *AC
Considered safe and one study demonstrated its immunostimulant effects.[354]

102. TARO (Colocasia esculenia) *AC
Top Recommended Edible Plant: Also in the Anticancer plant list for the same immunostimulant effect which causes the body to fight off tumor cells.[360]

103. TREE OF INDIA (Polyalthia longifolia) *AC
At least one study showed the leaf extract has immunostimulatory effects.[370]

104. TURKEY-TAIL MUSHROOM (Trametes versicolor) *AC
Top Recommended Holistic/Edible Mushroom: Just about all edible mushrooms, other than Button and Portabella, have more beta-Glucans, powerful immunostimulants and cancer fighters, and Turkey-Tail is no exception. Look for 100% pure dried powder, never fractions or mixtures which will be DILUTED with cheaper ingredients.[74][332]

105. VELVET LEAF (Cissampelos pareira) *AC
This plant has at least one study showing its immunostimulant effect.[377]

106. YAM (Dioscorea alata)
Top Recommended Edible Plant: Yams are one of the very few starchy root foods I recommend primarily because they have been shown to have a significant immunostimulatory effect.[69]

CONCLUSION
That's 462 plants (62 repeats, members in both lists) with proven anticancer or immunostimulant power which have been linked to the ability to prevent or even actively combat cancer.

A few are toxic, but I included them in the lists so you can see that even these plants have phytochemicals in them that science may eventually isolate and use as effective treatments for cancer.

Some plants in the Anticancer List are there only because of their immunostimulant power. It is important to remember that the human immune system is the first line of defense against any and all disease, including and especially cancer. There are many health professionals who believe that since the body contains many TRILLIONS of cells and that most organ systems constantly lose and replace cells, that during the average human lifespan there must be countless cell's that get DNA damage and if any one of them survives and divides, it could be the seed of cancer. Yet cancer was one of the rarest diseases prior to World War II, so the human immune system is very good at hunting these problem cells down and eradicating them; give the immune system everything it needs (that's the Big 43 Essential Nutrients) and the immune boosting plants and that is a very powerful first line of defense against cancer.

Many plants in the Anticancer Plant List make the list solely based on their ANTIOXIDANT content. There are over 1,100 tetraterpenoids alone and most of them are powerful antioxidants and many have been shown in numerous studies (like Lycopene) to have measurable anticancer power, some more so than others, but that doesn't take away from any antioxidant's positive power to help reduce the risk of and actively help combat cancer. In the next two chapters I will provide lists totaling 490 EDIBLE foods and spices loaded with proven anticancer compounds and most of them are powerful antioxidants bringing the total of discrete plant entries (not counting repeats) that can help you avoid and battle cancer to over 600: you would have to work hard to AVOID them all! And if you restrict your daily diet to ONLY FOODS from these lists then cancer doesn't stand a chance against that arsenal of powerful natural weapons.

The lists are not intended to overwhelm you but to give you choices and plenty of them. Many plants in this chapter will be hard to find in any form, but many are available as supplements or even on the shelf of your local grocery store right now. So how do you choose which ones to pursue? The two best kinds of study results involve plants that have shown anticancer effectiveness against a broad spectrum of different types of cancers and those that have shown SELECTIVE CYTOTOXICITY which means that the compounds in the plants target and kill cancer cells while leaving healthy cells virtually untouched. After that you definitely want to add every EDIBLE fruit. vegetable and spice that you can get your hands on and while you are at it, use these foods to REPLACE poor quality "non-functional" foods especially wheat (and all baked products) potatoes, rice and corn, all of which have very high Glycemic Index scores and are basically what I call "trash calories" that do nothing for you except increase your risk of Type II Diabetes and CANCER.

It doesn't mean that any of these plants will prevent you from getting cancer or cure it, but it does mean that each one will help and a diet consisting of only these plants will DRAMATICALLY REDUCE YOUR RISK OF CANCER AND CAN HELP DEFEAT IT.

This is a list of the phytonutrients with known anticancer properties and the edible plants that contain them. This list includes many more plants than just the ones specifically mentioned in the Anticancer, Immunostimulant and upcoming Antioxidant Plant Lists. Amounts are for milligrams per 100 gram serving and all foods are raw unless stated otherwise.

ACETOGENINS – Class of Flavonoids unique to species of Annona fruit trees: ANON, ATEMOYA, BULL'S HEART, CHERIMOYA, CUSTARD APPLE, POND APPLE, SOURSOP, SWEETSOP

ANTHOCYANIDIN – Category of Antioxidant Flavonoids: AÇAI 53.64mg, ACEROLA 22.55mg, ARCTIC BRAMBLE BERRY 89mg, BILBERRY 285.21mg, BLACK BEANS 44.52mg, BLACK CURRANT 157.78mg, BLACK PLUM 56.05mg, BLACKBERRY 99.95mg, BLACK RASPBERRY 686.79mg, BLUEBERRY 163.3mg, CHOKEBERRY 349.79mg, COCO PLUM 72.73mg, CONCORD GRAPE 120.1mg, CRANBERRY 104mg, EGGPLANT 85.69mg, ELDERBERRY 485.28mg, LINGONBERRY 40.15mg, MAQUI BERRY 88.52mg, RED RASPBERRY 48.63mg, RED CABBAGE 209.95mg, RADICCHIO 134.67mg, RADISHES 63.13mg, SERVICEBERRY 180.78mg, STRAWBERRY 27mg, SWEET CHERRY 31.98mg, TASMANIAN PEPPER 752.68mg, WILD RASPBERRY (Rubus moluccanus) 94.24mg[462]

APIGENIN – Flavonoid: CELERY SEED 78.65mg, CELERY HEARTS 19.1mg, CHINESE CELERY 24.02mg, KUMQUAT 21.87mg, MALABAR SPINACH (Basella) 62.2mg, PARSLEY (Dried) 4503mg[462]

ARCTIGENIN – Lignan: Some members of the Family Asteraceae (the Asters) including BURDOCK.[463]

BETA-GLUCANS – Oligosaccharides: BARLEY 86.1g, OATS 5.0g, AGARICUS BLAZEI 16.9g, BUTTON 7.5g, CHAGA 8.5g, ENOKI 21.0g, JUDAS EAR, MAITAKE 27.5g, PORTABELLA 7.2g, OYSTER 33.3g, REISHI 45.1g, SHIITAKE 27.4g, TURKEY-TAIL Mushrooms 40.4g.[332]

BETA-SITOSTEROL – Phytosterol: AVOCADO, NUTS, VEGETABLE OILS[460]

BETACYANIN – See BETALAINS

BETALAINS – Compounds found mostly in BEETS, but also SWISS CHARD[464]

BETULINIC ACID – Triterpenoid: ROSEMARY.[465]

CARVONE – Terpenoid: up to 70% of CARAWAY SEED OIL, 60% DILL SEED OIL, 60% MANDARIN ORANGE PEEL OIL, 50–80% SPEARMINT OIL[466]

CARYOPHELLENE – Sesquiterpenoid: Very common in spices and essential oils: BLACK CARAWAY 7.8%, CLOVE OIL 1.7–19.5%, HOPS 5.1–14.5%, BASIL 5.3–19.8%, OREGANO 4.9–15.7%, BLACK PEPPER 7.29%, LAVENDER OIL 4.62–7.55%, ROSEMARY 0.1–8.3%, CINNAMON 6.9–11.1%, YLANG-YLANG 3.1–10.7%[467]

CATECHIN – Flavan-3-ol: APRICOT 2mg/100g, BANANA 6.1mg, BLACK GRAPES 10.14mg, BLACK PLUM 17.55mg, BLACKBERRY 37.06mg, BLUEBERRY 5.29mg, CACAO (Baker's Unsweetened chocolate bars) 64.33mg, CAROB FLOUR 50.75mg, FAVA BEANS (Cooked) 8.16mg, JUJUBE 3.21mg, NECTARINE 2.98mg, PEACH 4.92mg, PECAN 7.24mg, PISTACHIO 3.57mg, STAR FRUIT, STRAWBERRY 3.11mg, SWEET

CHERRY 4.36mg, SWISS CHARD (Red leaf) 6.7mg, TEA (Green, brewed) 4.47mg[462]

CHICORIC ACID – Polyphenolic: Found in high concentrations in Chicory but also: ECHINACEA, DANDELION LEAVES, BASIL, LEMON BALM, AQUATIC PLANTS (i.e. LOTUS), ALGAE (i.e. KELP).[468]

CHLOROGENIC ACID – Polyphenolic acid ester: Present in high amounts in COFFEE but it is also in: DRIED PLUMS, EGGPLANT, PEACHES.[469]

CINEOL – Monoterpenoid: A.k.a. Eucalyptol; abundant in Eucalyptus but found in many spices and essential oils: WORMWOOD, TEA TREE (Melaleuca,) GALANGAL, BAY LAUREL, SPANISH SAGE, GINGER.[470]

CUCURBITACINS – Triterpenoids; Large group of compounds unique to Cucumbers and their kin: BITTER MELON, CANTALOUPE, CHAYOTE, CUCUMBER, INDIAN ZEHNERIA, PUMPKIN, SNAKE GOURD[471]

EGCG – Flavan-3-ol: Epigallocatechin-3-gallate, a powerful antioxidant found in high concentrations in GREEN TEA, but other plants contain it as well: BLACK GRAPES 2.81mg/100g, CAROB FLOUR 109.46mg, PECAN 2.3mg, TEA (Black, Brewed) 9.36mg, TEA (Green, brewed) 70.2mg[462]

ELLAGIC ACID – Phenolic: CRANBERRY, GRAPES, POMEGRANATE, RASPBERRY, STRAWBERRY, PECAN, PEACH, WALNUT.[472]

EPICATECHIN – Flavan-3-ol, APPLE JUICE (100% Pure) 4.71mg/100g, APRICOT 4.74mg, BLACK GRAPES 8.63mg, BLACK PLUM 2.44mg, BLACKBERRY 4.66mg, BULL'S HEART 5.63mg, CACAO (Baker's Unsweetened chocolate bars) 141.83mg, CRANBERRY 4.37mg, FAVA BEANS (Cooked) 7.82mg, NECTARINE 2.54mg, PEACH 2.34mg, RASPBERRY 3.52mg, RED DELICIOUS APPLE 9.83mg, RED WINE VINEGAR 2.2mg, STAR FRUIT, SWEET CHERRY 5mg, TEA (Black, Brewed) 2.13mg, TEA (Green, brewed) 8.33mg[462]

EPIGALLOCATECHIN – Flavan-3-ol: ALMONDS 2.59mg/100g, BLACK PLUM 13.06mg, FAVA BEANS (Cooked) 4.65mg, HAZELNUT 2.78mg, PECAN 5.63mg, PISTACHIO 2.05mg, TEA (Black, Brewed) 8.05mg, TEA (Green, brewed) 29.18mg[462]

FERULIC ACID – Organic Acid, common in most plants, but also found in: OLIVE, STAR FRUIT, and high bioavailability in ONIONS.[473]

GALLIC ACID – Precursor to METHYL GALLATE, EPIGALLOCATECHIN-3-GALLATE and EPIGALLOCATECHIN.

GENISTEIN – Isoflavone: Numerous studies have shown efficacy against a wide range of cancers. MODERATION IS ADVISED: COFFEE, KUDZU, FAVA BEANS. [474]

GLUCOSINOLATES – Major category of Phytonutrients that contain at least one sulfur atom. Subcategories are: Isothiocyanate Precursors, Organosulfides, Aglycones, and Indoles. The cruciferous vegetables like BROCCOLI, CAULIFLOWER, CABBAGE, ASPARAGUS, BRUSSELS SPROUTS, etc. as well as the Allium genus including ONIONS, GARLIC, SHALLOTS, and LEEKS are all excellent sources of various forms of glucosinolates.[475]

INDOLE-3-CARBINOL – Glucosinolate: BROCCOLI, KALE, BRUSSELS SPROUTS, CABBAGE, CAULIFLOWER, COLLARD GREENS[476]

INULIN – Polysaccharide/Dietary Fiber: CHICORY, ONION, BANANAS, GARLIC, ASPARAGUS, JERUSALEM ARTICHOKE[477]

KAEMPFEROL – Antioxidant Flavonol: Kaempferol is all or nothing; either present in micrograms or significant amounts: ARUGULA 34.89mg/100g, BOK CHOY 4.33mg, BROCCOLI 7.84mg, CAPERS (Canned) 131.34mg, CHIA SEED (raw) 12.3mg, CHIVES 10mg, COLLARD GREENS 8.74mg, CRESS (Lepidium sativum) 13mg, DOCK (Rumex) 10.3mg, DRUMSTICK

TREE (leaves, raw) 5.95mg, ENDIVE 10.1mg, GOJI BERRY (Dried) 6.2mg, PINECONE GINGER 33.6mg, KALE 46.8mg, LOVAGE (leaves) 7mg, MUSTARD GREENS 38.3mg, NEW ZEALAND SPINACH 15.75mg, SAFFRON 205.48mg, SPINACH 6.38mg, SWISS CHARD (Red leaf) 9.2mg, TURNIP GREENS 11.87mg, WATERCRESS (Nasturtium officinale) 23.03mg, WELSH ONION (A. fistulosum) 24.95mg[462]

LUPEOL – Triterpenoid: MANGO, DANDELION.[478]

LUTEOLIN – Flavone: MEXICAN OREGANO, Dried 1028mg/100g, SAGE (Fresh) 15.7mg, CELERY SEED 762.4mg, CHINESE CELERY 34.87mg, THYME, Fresh 45.25mg, JUNIPER BERRY 69.05mg, PIMENTO 10.36mg, QUEEN ANNE'S LACE (Leaves) 34.1mg, RADICCHIO 37.98mg.[462]

METHYL GALLATE – Organic Acid Ester: Can occur in foods high in Gallic Acid: OLIVES, HOG PLUM, STRAWBERRIES, GRAPES, TEA, BANANAS, CLOVES, RED WINE VINEGAR[479]

OLEIC ACID – Monounsaturated Omega-9 fatty acid: The majority of OLIVE OIL (as triglycerides of Oleic acid), 59–75% of PECAN OIL, 61% of CANOLA OIL, 36–67% of PEANUT OIL, 60% of MACADAMIA OIL, 20–80% SUNFLOWER OIL, 15–20% GRAPE SEED OIL, SEA BUCKTHORN OIL, and SESAME SEED OIL, 14% of POPPYSEED OIL, 22.18% of the fats from DURIAN fruit.[480]

OLIGOSACCHARIDES – Carbohydrates; A large class of complex sugars some with immunostimulant power: AVOCADO, CASHEW, NONI, ALOE, RADISHES, AGAVE, BANANAS, ONIONS, CHICORY ROOT, GARLIC, ASPARAGUS, JICAMA, LEEKS, BARLEY, JERUSALEM ARTICHOKE

PALMITIC ACID – Saturated Fatty Acid: Highest in cold-expeller extra virgin PALM OIL, COCONUT OIL, PEANUT OIL[481]

PECTIN – Polysaccharide, Fiber: One study in Chernobyl found that increased Pectin helped reduce the amount of radioactive heavy metal contamination in foods from getting into the body: PEAR, APPLE, GUAVA, QUINCE, PLUM, GOOSEBERRY, CITRUS[482]

PERILLYL ALCOHOL – Monoterpenoid: LEMONGRASS, SAGE, LAVENDER, PEPPERMINT[483]

PHYSALINS – Phytonutrients found only in the Physalis genus (and a few closely related genera) along with Withanolides and Withaphysalins: CAPE GOOSEBERRY, SUNBERRY[96][352]

PHYTOESTROGENS – Major class of plant compounds that can mimic mammalian estrogen. They have shown efficacy against certain forms of cancer, but could exacerbate others: TEMPEH, FLAXSEED, SESAME SEEDS, FENUGREEK, OATS, BARLEY, BEANS, LENTILS, YAMS, ALFALFA, MUNG BEANS, APPLE, CARROT, POMEGRANATE, WHEAT GERM, CELERY, RICE BRAN, KUDZU, COFFEE, LICORICE, MINT, FENNEL, ANISE[484]

PICEATANNOL – Stilbenoid: GRAPE, PASSION FRUIT, WHITE TEA[485]

PIPERINE - : BLACK PEPPER, LONG PEPPER, JAVA PEPPER[461]

QUERCETIN – Flavonoid: CAPERS, Canned 173mg/100g, DILL 55mg, CILANTRO 53mg, ONION, Red 32mg, RADICCHIO 32mg, KALE 23mg, WATERCRESS 30mg, CRANBERRY 15mg, LINGONBERRY 13mg, PLUMS, Black 12mg[462]

RUTIN – Flavonoid: CAPERS 332mg, BLACK OLIVE 45mg, BUCKWHEAT (whole grain flour) 36mg, ASPARAGUS 23mg, BLACK RASPBERRY 19mg, RED RASPBERRY 11mg, BUCKWHEAT, GROATS 9mg, PLUM 6mg, BLACK CURRANT 5mg, BLACKBERRY 4mg, TOMATO (Cherry) 3mg, DRIED PLUM 2mg.[462]

SQUALENE – Triterpenoid: SHARK LIVER OIL (not recommended), AMARANTH SEED, RICE BRAN, WHEAT GERM, OLIVES[486]
SULFORAPHANE – Isothiocyanate: Found in cruciferous vegetables including: BROCCOLI, BRUSSELS SPROUTS, CABBAGE[487]
TARAXASTEROL – Phytosterol: CHICORY, DANDELION ROOT[147]
URSOLIC ACID – Triterpenoid: APPLE, BASIL, BILBERRY, CRANBERRY, DRIED PLUM, ELDER FLOWER, HAWTHORN, LAVENDER, OREGANO, PEPPERMINT, ROSEMARY, THYME[488]
WITHANOLIDES – See PHYSALINS.[96]
WITHAPHYSALINS – See PHYSALINS.[96]

CONCLUSION

These lists have provided over 333 distinct plants that have known anticancer and/or immunostimulant properties or powerful antioxidant content that can definitely help prevent and even combat cancer. Many are already in the Anticancer Plants List and/or Immunostimulant Plants Lists of the previous chapter and many will appear again in the lists of plants high in antioxidants in the coming chapter as well.

Plants/Foods with More than One Effective Phytonutrient

All Edible Mushrooms	Caraway	Macadamia
Almond	Carob	Mint
Apple	Celery	Nectarine
Apricot	Chinese Celery	Oats
Asparagus	Chicory	Onion
Avocado	Clove	Oregano
Banana	Coffee	Peach
Basil	Collard Greens	Pecan
Bilberry	Cranberry	Pistachio
Black Currant	Dandelion	Pomegranate
Black Pepper	Dill	Radicchio
Black Plum	Dried Plum	Radish
Black Raspberry	Eggplant	Raspberry
Blackberry	Elderberry	Red Wine Vinegar
Blueberry	Endive	Rosemary
Broccoli	Fava Beans	Sesame
Brussels Sprouts	Garlic	Star Fruit
Buckwheat	Green Tea	Strawberry
Bull's Heart	Hazelnut*	Sweet Cherry
Cabbage	Kale	Swiss Chard
Cacao	Kudzu	Thyme
Cape Gooseberry*	Lavender	Watercress
Capers	Lingonberry	Wheat Germ

* Cape Gooseberry for the Physalins and Withaphysalins, Hazelnuts also contain beta-Sitosterol

Many of these foods are featured in "Getting the Big 43 Essential Nutrients The Natural Way Vol. 1" for their essential nutrient content as well.

There are many plants, including edible foods, spices and holistic herbs that have "anticancer" properties. And this is admittedly a very indefinite term: what does it mean to have an "anticancer" property? Some plants may be very significant in their ability to PREVENT cancer – a very good property since the best defense against any disease is not to get it in the first place. But many such plants have shown inconclusive results in combating existing cancer. So they can prevent it, but they can't help you to overcome it once it has a foothold. I would argue that most of these plants, especially edible foods, certainly won't do any harm after the cancer has started, but you would definitely want to add foods, spices and holistic herbs from the lists of the two preceding chapters that have shown the ability to actively combat cancer especially those that have shown positive results against the cell line you have. Since most testing concentrates on a small minority of all identified cell lines, then the next best choices are: plants that have shown broad spectrum power against many different types of cancer or those that have shown strong anticancer power against other types of cancers of the same organ.

Again, this is not about a cure: it is about AUGMENTING your doctor's efforts and many plants in the preceding lists have been shown to actually ASSIST chemotherapy by making the cancerous cells more susceptible to it; and that would be yet another example of an "anticancer" property.

The immune system is the human body's first line of defense against ALL possible invaders including cancer, even though cancer is technically not an invader, but DNA-damaged (i.e. mutated) cells of your own body. But, the immune system can detect them and destroy them and that is why many of the plants in the Immunostimulant Plant list have the anticancer property: they crank up the immune system to attack the cancerous cells. But you can't stomp on the gas pedal of your car if it has no oil in the engine either. That would permanently destroy the engine. And you can't ask your immune system to go into high gear if the body does not have everything it needs to build more white blood cells or defensive molecules like Interleukin, if it doesn't have all of the basic building blocks necessary to get this done: and those are all of the members of the "Big 43" essential nutrients.

THE ANTICANCER DIET

This diet combines the best of many different diets that have been advocated throughout the years by many different well respected health professionals. Some of these diets may well be extremely effective in their original layout, but since some of them advocate certain foods like raw beef liver, I have selected the best features from each while omitting these other questionable items. There is little doubt that raw beef liver is a true Superfood; it is loaded with many vitamins and minerals and other constituents that represent not only the Big 43 in respectable amounts, but it also brings far too much saturated fat and cholesterol and both of these are a significant concern to total overall health. Also, all members of the Big 43 that beef liver provides can also be obtained from well chosen plant foods anyway.

1. GET THE BIG 43 – You must give your body what it needs to be as strong as possible to help fight off disease. Even so, you should ASK YOUR DOCTOR BEFORE YOU LOAD UP ON THE BIG 43 ESPECIALLY FROM SUPPLEMENTS. See "Getting the Big 43 Essential Nutrients The Natural Way, Vol.1" for all you need to know: recommended amounts, best food sources, etc.

2. ELIMINATE ALL JUNK/FAST FOOD – This includes all foods high in trash calories and the main culprits are: ALCOHOL, SODA, WHEAT (virtually ALL BAKED goods including 100% Whole wheat bread and any other types such as Barley, Rye, etc,) RICE, CORN and POTATOES.

3. LOAD UP ON ANTIOXIDANTS – The only problem with this is that very few supplements have been shown to be effective. This is because the processing of the compound into the pills causes it to become DEPLETED of its antioxidant power. Beta-carotene pills DO NOT WORK, but all Natural Whole Food sources including Carrots, Butternut Squash, Sweet Potatoes, etc, have been shown in studies to be very effective for their antioxidant power. There are thousands of antioxidants, not just the famous ones like Lycopene, beta-Carotene, Lutein and Zeaxanthin and most are very powerful nutrients that the body recognizes and puts to work cleaning up tissues of toxic metabolic waste by-products. But this is certainly not the only thing these compounds do; many have other functions in the body as well. Beta-Carotene and many other Carotenoids can be converted by the liver into Retinol – true Vitamin A – on demand. And while it is in the form of beta-Carotene, it is 25 times more potent as an antioxidant than Vitamin C.

Many people are megadosing on Vitamin C hoping to cash in on its "Free Radical Scavenging" power. Unfortunately, they are not reaping those benefits at all. By taking a lot of Vitamin C, say 2500mg, the Kidneys notice the excess and begin to pull it out of the bloodstream, so it won't be there for long. But 100mg of beta-Carotene which has the same antioxidant power could be left to wander in the blood neutralizing oxidants.

But not all antioxidants are the same. Some are much more powerful than others, and each one has its own affinity: which oxidants it is better at neutralizing. Also different organs in the body have their preferences as well. While the liver likes them all, the skin likes beta-Carotene, the bones like Lycopene and the eyes like beta-Carotene as well as Lutein, Zeaxanthin and many others. Because of this there is no way to establish an RDA. Which ones should be included when there are so many and science is discovering new ones and new health benefits of known ones all the time?

The best approach is to load up on the antioxidants because CANCER happens to CREATE and PREFER an OXIDANT-RICH environment. So if your diet is relatively poor in antioxidants then your entire body is an OXIDANT-RICH environment and that's what CANCER LIKES. Loading up on the antioxidants GREATLY REDUCES THE RISK OF MOST FORMS OF CANCER and they also REDUCE ITS GROWTH, PROLIFERATION and SPREAD.

Common Foods Highest Antioxidant Density Per Calorie

FOOD	ORAC	O/cal	O/g	Oz.	Cal
1. Cranberries	9090	196.08	90.90	3.5	46
2. Black Plums	7581	164.02	75.81	5.8	76
3. Strawberries	4302	132.57	43.02	5	46
4. Dark chocolate	49944	101.14	499.44	4	560
5. Artichokes (cooked)	4760	91.49	47.60	4	59
6. Red Delicious Apple	4275	82.04	42.75	4.4	65
7. Blueberries	4669	81.94	46.69	5.2	84
8. Arugula	1904	75.57	19.04	0.7	5
9. Asparagus (cooked)	1644	73.41	16.44	6.3	40
10. Black beans (can)	6416	70.92	64.16	8.5	218
11. Spinach	1513	67.40	15.13	1.1	7
12. Alfalfa Sprouts	1510	64.21	15.10	1.2	8
13. Bean Sprouts	1510	64.21	15.10	1.2	8
14. Lentils	7282	62.83	72.82	7	230
15. Broccoli (cooked)	2160	61.24	21.60	5.5	55
16. Blackeye Peas	4343	56.57	43.43	8.5	185
17. Beets (canned)	1776	56.51	17.76	5.5	49
18. Swiss Chard	1108	55.64	11.08	6.2	35
19. Pomegranate	4479	53.79	44.79	6.1	144
20. Grapefruit (red)	1640	51.03	16.40	9	82
21. Figs	3383	45.36	33.83	3.5	74
22. Brussels sprouts*	1330	37.03	13.30	5.5	56
23. Cabbage (boiled)	856	36.75	8.56	5.3	35
24. Kale	1770	35.42	17.70	1.2	17
25. Dried Plums	8059	33.34	80.59	6.1	418
26. Celery	552	32.22	5.52	3.5	17
27. Cauliflower (cook)	739	31.79	7.39	4.4	29
28. Lettuce (Iceberg)	438	31.04	4.38	2.5	10
29. Tangerine	1627	30.90	16.27	6.9	103
30. Bell Peppers	935	29.71	9.35	3.25	29
31. Pecans	17940	25.56	179.40	3	597
32. Button Mushrooms	691	25.55	6.91	3	23
33. Grapes (black)	1746	25.23	17.46	5.3	104
34. Green beans (can)	290	24.41	2.90	4.75	16
35. Tomato (cooked)	423	23.61	4.23	6.3	32
36. Sweet Potato*	2115	23.32	21.15	7	180
37. Apricot	1110	22.68	11.10	4.9	68
38. Mango	1300	21.59	13.00	5.8	99
39. Walnuts (English)	13541	20.98	135.41	1	183
40. Guava	1422	20.88	14.22	5.8	112

Antioxidant ORAC Densities per Calorie (cont.)

FOOD	ORAC	O/cal	O/g	Oz.	Cal
41. Pineapple	943	18.68	9.43	5.8	83
42. Leeks	569	17.64	5.69	3.5	32
43. Carrots	697	17.10	6.97	4.5	52
44. Pumpkin (canned)	483	14.19	4.83	8.6	83
45. Kiwi	862	14.14	8.62	6.25	108
46. Onions (Sweet)	614	14.00	6.14	7.4	92
47. Pistachios	7675	13.60	76.75	3	480
48. Avocado	1922	12.03	19.22	5.3	240
49. Cucumber	140	11.66	1.40	4.7	16
50. Raisins (seedless)	3406	11.27	34.06	3.5	300

* Brussels sprouts are steamed, Sweet Potato is baked w/skin.

These are the top 50 foods by ORAC Score per calorie (O/cal) and though the ORAC – Oxygen Radical Absorption Capacity – score is now considered obsolete, no matter how the content of antioxidants is measured, since they are all different, there is no way to come up with an "Absolute" measuring system anyway.

"O/g" is ORAC score per gram. You will find that all of the seeds and nuts have very high antioxidant densities per gram meaning that a much smaller amount by weight is required to deliver a lot of antioxidant power. However, this is probably more useful to NASA, where the weight of the food is a big concern. "Oz." indicates a "typical" serving size and "Cal" indicates how many calories that serving brings. Some extremely low calorie foods rank very high in the list like Alfalfa Sprouts.

How this table works is simple. Choose a food, say #4 - Dark Chocolate. In order to get as much antioxidant power as any amount of it, say 280 calories (2 ounces,) then you would have to eat more calories than that of any food below it in the list. That means that Cranberries, Black Plums, Strawberries and Red Delicious Apples (as well as Dark Chocolate) are ALL on my regular menu and you should include them in your daily snacks and desserts as well.

The greatest antioxidant densities are found in the dried and powdered spices. Not only do they have astronomical ORAC Scores, but they also have very powerful phytonutrients in them many of which have been shown to possess extraordinary health benefits including many that can actively COMBAT CANCER.

THE SPICE RACK – THE ANTIOXIDANT POWERHOUSE
Allspice (100,400 ground), **Basil** (61,063 dried, 4,805 fresh), **Black Pepper** (34,053), **Cayenne Pepper** (19,671 ground), **Chili Powder** (23,636), **Cilantro** (5,141 fresh), **Cinnamon** (131,420), **Cloves** (290,283), **Cumin** (50,372), **Curry Powder** (48,504), **Dill Weed** (4,392 fresh), **Garlic** (6,665 dried; 5,708 fresh), **Ginger Root** (39,041 ground,14,840 raw), **Lemon Balm** (5,997 fresh), **Marjoram** (92,310 dried), **Nutmeg** (69,640 ground), **Oregano** (175,295 dried; 13,970 fresh), **Paprika** (21,932), **Parsley** (73,670 dried), **Peppermint Leaves** (160,820 dried, 13,978 fresh),

Rosemary (165,280 dried; 11,070 fresh), **Saffron** (whole, 20,580),**Sage** (119,929 dried; 32,004 fresh), **Savory** (9,465 fresh), **Star Anise** (11,300), **Tarragon** (15,542 fresh), **Thyme** (157,380 dried, 27,426 fresh), **Turmeric** (127,068 dried), **Vanilla Bean Spice** (122,400 dried), **Yellow Mustard Seed** (29,257)[2]

That's 30 spices and most can be found at any well stocked grocery store. Most dried spices have immense ORAC scores because most of the water has been removed and water makes up about 85% of all plant matter except for seeds which are naturally desiccated and waiting to absorb water like a sponge in order to sprout; so they are already naturally dehydrated and concentrated and loaded with antioxidants. Dried fruits like raisins and prunes also have much higher ORAC scores for the same reason.[2]

If a doctor told me today that I have cancer, I would run to the grocery store and buy nothing but the foods with these highest concentrations of antioxidants and eat them all day long and I would cook with heavy applications of as many spices as possible (I happen to do this anyway, but you get the idea.) In addition to that I would also take Astaxanthin. It is a triterpenoid and it is roughly SIX THOUSAND TIMES more potent than Vitamin C. To put that in perspective, a 4mg gelcap has the antioxidant power of TWENTY-FOUR THOUSAND MILLIGRAMS of Vitamin C. That's FORTY-EIGHT 500mg Vitamin C pills worth of antioxidant power in a single Astaxanthin pill. So put away the BB gun and pick up the BAZOOKA of antioxidants.

RECOMMENDED ASTAXANTHIN SUPPLEMENT
==

MANUFACTURER: SPRING VALLEY
PRODUCT NAME: ASTAXANTHIN 4MG, 30 GELCAPS
This store-bought Astaxanthin product is a natural source extract taken from a species of red algae which makes it a quality product and recommended over synthetic forms. Be VERY CAREFUL with ASTAXANTHIN: it is so STRONG that it can actually DEPLETE your IMMUNE SYSTEM. I take it once or twice a week. But if diagnosed with Cancer, I would take at least 4mg per day and take a spread of immunostimulants to compensate.

77 MORE FOODS WITH HIGH ORAC SCORES
Lingonberry, (20300), **Maqui Berry** (19850), **Black Raspberry** (19220), **Bael Fruit** (17933), **Chokeberry** (16062), **Serviceberry** (**Saskatoon Berry**, **Juneberry**, 15000), **Elderberry** (14697), **Golden Raisins** (Seedless, 10450), **Black Chia Seeds** (Raw, 9800), **Hazelnuts** (9645), **Black Currants** (7957), **Black Crowberries** (7890), **Wild Bilberries** (7570), **White Chia Seeds** (Raw, 7000), **Burdock Root** (Raw, 6747), **Mulberries** (6130), **Blackberries** (5905), **Red Raspberries** (5065), **Black Quinoa** (Raw, 4800), **Chestnuts** (4670), **Sea Buckthorn Berries** (4580), **Almonds** (4454), **Red Quinoa** (Raw, 3900), **Deglet Noor Dates** (3895), **Cape Gooseberries** (**Inca Berries**, **Golden Berries**,

3874), **Sweet Cherries** (3747), **Tamarind** (3500), **Peanut Butter** (3432), **Red Currants** (3387), **Gooseberries** (3332), **Goji Berry** (3290), **Quinoa** (White, Uncooked, 3200), **Peanuts** (Raw, All Varieties, 3166), **Red Cabbage** (Boiled, 3145), **Kalamata Olives** (3130), **Cloudberry** (a.k.a. Knotberries, 2530), **Mangosteen** (2510), **Red Leaf Lettuce** (Raw, 2426), **Medjool Dates** (2387), **Rowan Berries** (2360), **Purple Cauliflower** (Cooked, 2210), **Oranges** (All Varieties, 2103), **Chives** (Raw, 2094), **Savoy Cabbage** (Boiled, 2050), **Cashews** (1948), **Beet Greens** (Raw, 1946), **Peaches** (1922), **Red Grapes** (1837), **Navel Oranges** (1819), **Lacinato Kale** (**Dinosaur, Tuscan, Black Kale**, Cooked, 1773), **Radishes** (Raw, 1750), **Black Grapes** (1746), **Oatmeal** (Old Fashioned Oats, Uncooked, 1708), **Macadamia Nuts** (1695), **Mandarins** (1627), **Red Onions** (Raw, 1521), **Jaboticaba Fruit** (1511), **Soursop** (1451), **Bibb Butter Lettuce** (Boston, Raw, 1423), **Brazil Nuts** (Unblanched, 1419), **Romanesco Cauliflower** (**Broccoflower, Green Cauliflower**, Cooked, 1387), **Safflower Oil** (1380), **Lemons** (1346), **Raw Agave** (1294), **Ground Flaxseed** (1130), **Coconut Oil** (1070), **Romaine Lettuce** (Raw, 1017), **Green Olives** (1010)

4. LOAD UP ON DIETARY FIBER – Try to get 100% RDA of this important member of the Big 43 from Natural Whole Foods first and ONLY USE A SUPPLEMENT with meals to make up the difference for the day. It has been shown to reduce the risk of digestive tract cancers and it doesn't matter if you do not have colon cancer, improving digestive tract health means improving your ability to absorb ALL NUTRIENTS from the foods, spices and holistic herbs that you consume. Some of the best sources of Dietary Fiber (the "good" kind) are: CACAO, BLACK BEANS, LENTILS, DRIED PLUMS (a.k.a. Prunes, but don't let that turn you off, they are amazingly good for your health) and CHICKPEAS.[71]

5. FRESH JUICES – This is part of the Gerson Diet, a well respected natural cancer therapy. Most commercial juices are made from high speed expellers that heat up the product to the point that it begins to damage much of the nutritional content including the vitamins and the antioxidants. You should eat whole raw fruits as the only snack items for the day and make fresh juice as the only drinks aside from herbal teas. And don't forget the vegetables; this is the true power of drinking an average of 13 glasses a day (the Gerson Diet protocol.)

6. COTTAGE CHEESE and ALA – This is the cornerstone of the Budwig Diet. Dr. Budwig found that consuming certain types of Saturated Fat (the Cottage Cheese, high in sulfur-containing amino acids) along with certain unsaturated fatty acids found in plants (the ALA – Alpha-Linoleic Acid) had a significant anticancer and anti-inflammatory effect. Most plant Omega-6 fatty acids like CLA – Conjugated Linoleic Acid (found in Borage Oil) and Punicic Acid (unique to Pomegranates) have been proven to be potent anti-inflammatory agents. Mix ground Chia or Flax seed in one serving (i.e. 6 to 8 oz.) of Cottage Cheese and add spices like Turmeric, Ginger, and Black Pepper.[17]

7. CONCENTRATE ON THE FOODS WITH PROVEN IMMUNE BOOSTING and ANTICANCER PROPERTIES -

Edible Plants with Anticancer and/or Immunostimulant Power

Açai Berry	Custard Apple	Oats
Acerola	Dates	Okra
Alfalfa	Dragon Fruit	Olives
Amaranth	Durian	Onion
Amla	Eggplant	Otaheite Gooseberry
Asparagus	Elderberry	Papaya
Bael	Endive	Passion Fruit
Barley Grass	Fennel	Peanuts
Beet	Goji Berry	Pigeon Pea
Bignay	Gotu Kola	Pineapple
Bitter Melon	Governor's Plum	Pink Wampee
Black Currant	Grapes	Pomegranate
Black Myrobalan	Green Peas	Pomelo
Bok Choy	Guava	Portabella Mushroom
Borage	Hog Plum	Pumpkin
Bottle Gourd	Jaboticaba	Pumpkin Seed
Breadfruit	Jackfruit	Radish
Broccoli	Jamaican Cherry	Rambutan
Bull's Heart	Jujube	Schisandra
Burdock	Jute	Sea Buckthorn
Button Mushroom	Karandas	Seaside Plum
Cabbage	Kudzu	Shallot
Canistel	Langsat	Snake Gourd
Cantaloupe	Lemon	Sour Orange
Cape Gooseberry	Lettuce	Soursop
Capers	Lime	Star Apple
Carrot	Luffa	Star Fruit
Cashew	Lychee	Strawberry
Celery	Malay Apple	Sugar Cane
Chayote	Mamey	Sunberry
Cherimoya	Mango	Tamarind
Chico Sapodilla	Mangosteen	Tomato
Chicory	Marang	Wampee
Chinese Lantern	Miracle Fruit	Wild Raspberry
Chinese Strawberry	Mulberry	Yam
Coconut	Mustard Greens	Yard-Long Bean

That's 108 edible fruits and vegetables with PROVEN anticancer and/or immunostimulant powers. Some will be much harder to find but even canned Asparagus and Pineapple are staples of most grocery stores and many of these foods are available in the fresh produce section as well (and are highly preferred.)

8. CRANK UP THE SPICES – These are powerhouses loaded with many phytonutrients in high concentrations (hence their strong aromas and flavors) and many of them are currently under investigation and demonstrating extraordinary health promoting properties.

While most folks (in the U.S.) only cook with a pinch of salt and pepper, that is a CULTURAL thing. Spices have very powerful phytonutrients in high concentrations including the high antioxidant scores, just one level teaspoon of clove powder (about 2 grams) brings the equivalent antioxidant power of almost TWO POUNDS of raw carrots, not to mention the PROVEN anticancer and immunostimulant properties amongst many other health benefits that the spices also bring to the table.

Culinary Spices and Misc. Foods with Anticancer and/or Immunostimulant Properties

Agave	Cloves	Mustard Seed
Amaranth	Coriander	Oregano
Anise	Curry Leaf	Parsley
Annatto	Fennel Seed	Patchouli
Basil	Flax Seed	Rosemary
Betel Pepper	Garlic	Safflower
Black Pepper	Ginger	Sage
Cacao(1)	Indian Patchouli	Sarsaparilla
Capers	Job's Tears(2)	Sesame(3)
Caraway	Lemon Grass	Spirulina
Cardamom	Licorice	Taro
Chamomile	Long Pepper	Turmeric
Cilantro	Marjoram	Vanilla

(1) Pure Unsweetened Baker's Dark Chocolate
(2) Job's Tears can be found as 100% whole grain flour for baking.
(3) Sesame Seed Butter, a.k.a. "Tahini" is the best choice

That's 39 spices and miscellaneous foods with PROVEN anticancer and/or immunostimulant powers that you can add to your cooking and most are common and can be found in most well-stocked grocery stores.

8. GREEN LEAFY VEGETABLES – There is plenty of evidence that these plants reduce the risk of most of the BIG SEVEN MODERN DEADLY EPIDEMIC PLAGUES: High Blood Pressure, High Cholesterol, Cardiovascular Disease, Type II Diabetes, Alzheimer's disease, Stroke and CANCER. The leafy vegetables like LETTUCE, CABBAGE, ARUGULA, BARLEY GRASS, KALE, SPINACH, COLLARD GREENS, MUSTARD GREENS, SWISS CHARD, BEET GREENS, TURNIP GREENS, etc are all loaded with Chlorophyll which is a potent liver detoxifier that can definitely help reduce the risk of liver cancer. Try to eat at least two cups per day, cooked or preferably raw. Add more servings each day by juicing them.

9. THE CRUCIFEROUS VEGETABLES – Numerous studies have shown that the plants loaded with glucosinolates (sulfur-containing compounds) are also excellent at combating the Big Seven Modern Deadly Epidemic Plagues. CABBAGE and BROCCOLI should be on the daily menu, but CAULIFLOWER, ASPARAGUS,

COLLARD GREENS, BRUSSELS SPROUTS, HORSERADISH, CRESS, MUSTARD (seeds and greens), KALE, CHINESE BROCCOLI, CABBAGE, SAVOY CABBAGE, KOHLRABI, BOK CHOY, BROCCOFLOWER, BROCCOLI ROMANESCO, WILD BROCCOLI, KOMATSUNA, MIZUNA, RAPINI (Rabe Broccoli), CHOY SUM (Flowering cabbage), NAPA CABBAGE, TURNIP (root and greens), RUTABAGA, SIBERIAN KALE, CANOLA (Rapeseed), WRAPPED HEART MUSTARD CABBAGE, TATSOI, WILD ARUGULA, ARUGULA (Rocket), FIELD PEPPERWEED, MACA, WATERCRESS, RADISH, DAIKON, WASABI should be included in your weekly diet as well as fresh SHALLOTS, LEEKS, ONIONS and GARLIC.

10. UNREFINED OILS – Almost all store-bought oils are refined: they have been overheated and even distilled (evaporated and recondensed) in order to purify the oil and remove the taste and odor of the original raw oil as much as possible. This also removes almost all of their phytonutrients and leaves them nothing but raw CALORIES with no nutritional compounds left in them. The best raw oils (unrefined, i.e. cold-pressed extra virgin) are in order: COCONUT, OLIVE, SESAME, SAFFLOWER, SUNFLOWER, and CANOLA. One teaspoon per day of COD LIVER OIL is also a must for the Vitamin A (90% RDA,) Vitamin D3 (113% RDA) and the DHA and EPA Omega-3 Fatty Acids (total 888mg of both) it brings.[7] Hydrogenated Oils – ARTIFICIAL ANIMAL FATS cooked up in a test tube – ARE TOXIC and those that get past the liver (which treats them like the TOXINS that they are) can DESTROY cell membranes which in turn increases the risk of ALL of the Big Seven Modern Deadly Epidemic Plagues. Read the Ingredients labels and avoid ALL products that have "hydrogenated" or "hydrolyzed" (similar process) oils of any kind in them. The healthy powerful oils are not on the menu for making fried foods: those are definitely NOT good for your health. You can sneak these in to home made Oil and Vinegar dressing, add them to Sour Cream (not the best food on Earth, but it is compared to mayonnaise and its kin; store-bought dips and creamy salad dressings, all made from raw eggs which are TOXIC) and home made Hummus.

11. TEA – But, don't stop at GREEN TEA, many of the plants in the Anticancer Plants and the Immunostimulants Plants lists are available as bulk dried powder for making herbal teas which are highly recommended as well.

12. STEAM INSTEAD OF BOIL, REDUCE COOKING HEAT AND TIME – Overcooked foods have reduced nutritional content because heat destroys molecules like Vitamin C, and can severely deplete many forms of antioxidants especially the tetraterpenoids like beta-Carotene (carrots and most other orange vegetables,) Lutein and Zeaxanthin (both found in the highest amounts in Kale, but present in most leafy greens.) The easy rule to remember is: the closer your plant foods are to raw; the better.

13. ADD THOSE BETA-GLUCANS – Numerous studies across the globe have proven that these compounds are powerful natural immunostimulants and cancer fighters. Most of the phytonutrients in these discussions are present in milligrams (1mg = 1/1000th of a gram) and some are only present in micrograms (1/1,000,000[th] of a gram) but ½ cup of Old fashioned oatmeal contains a whopping 5,400mg of Beta-Glucans, that's almost a fifth of an ounce or to be very clear: they comprise around 13% of the total mass of that ½ cup of Oatmeal. That is NOT a "trace" constituent, but rather a MAJOR component which is why I highly recommend oatmeal as the ONLY breakfast cereal for the rest of your life. And don't forget the edible mushrooms either. One cup of white Button Mushrooms brings about 23 calories and contains 6370mg (almost ¼ oz) of the beta-Glucans. It is by far the highest concentration per calorie of any readily available and inexpensive food. Because these beta-Glucans could be damaged by cooking, the mushrooms should be sliced raw into your lunch salad, and you can also make "raw Oatmeal" by mixing it with the desired amount of water and then placing it into the refrigerator overnight. [15][74]

14. DETOXIFICATION AND ANTI-INFLAMMATORY HERBS – Although neither is a specific topic of this volume of The Natural Way series, they are both critical to success. The Chlorophylls in the green leafy vegetables help the liver to detoxify as does Artichoke Leaf Extract available as a supplement from many vendors. Sticking to natural fruit and vegetable juices made fresh daily and kept in tightly sealed glass containers in the refrigerator ensures that you are getting plenty of liquids which helps the kidneys detoxify as well.

15. SUPERIOR "IDEAL" COMPLETE PROTEIN – This means FISH. Tuna, Cod, and Pollock in particular make up three of the four best sources of Protein per calorie and all three have nearly ideal ratios of the Nine Essential Amino Acids that the body cannot manufacture and that must come from foods. Five to seven ounces of Tuna will cover your needs for all of these amino acids easily and keep you away from eating excess protein which is a very dirty burning fuel that clogs up the cells with those metabolic waste by-products that the antioxidants have to clean up.

16. ADD ANTICANCER and IMMUNOSTIMULANT MEDICINAL HERBS – While there are many holistic herbs that are very hard to find in any form, many plants from the anticancer and immune stimulant lists can be found in supplement form from at least one manufacturer. Several are very well known in the holistic medicinal circles for powers other than anticancer and/or immunostimulants, but that should not deter you from trying them out. The studies have been done either directly on the plants in those lists or they have been done on other species that contain similar or exactly the same phytochemicals. Many of these plants are well-known in traditional herbal systems like Traditional Chinese Medicine or the ancient Ayurvedic practices of India for their immunostimulant and anticancer properties.

Read the labels and make certain that the manufacturer is not adding nonsense fillers or manufactured chemicals. Some store-bought dietary supplements are actually adding things like sugar (i.e. maltodextrose,) artificial colors, and so on. Most companies do NOT do this these days, but it is always wise to check. Also check the amounts of the actual plant present in each pill. Some well known medicinal plants are now sold based on a specific phytonutrient's amount such as "2% Corosolic Acid." This is fine as long as the content is NOT A FRACTION (partial extract,) but the "full spectrum" extract (all of the plant's contents are present.)

HOLISTIC HERBS AVAILABLE IN SUPPLEMENT FORM

Agrimony	Echinacea	Mimosa
Aloe	Eleuthero	Neem
Andrographis	Epimedium	Noni
Angelica	Eucalyptus	Oregon Grape Root
Ashitaba	Evening Primrose	Pau D'arco
Astragalus	Five-Leaf Chaste Tree	Red Clover
Barberry	Fo-Ti	Red Sorrel
Birch	Frankincense	Reishi Mushroom
Bishop's Weed	Galangal	Rhodiola
Blessed Thistle	Gardenia	Rooibos
Boneset	Ginkgo Biloba	Rose
Borage	Ginseng	Sarsaparilla
Burdock	Gotu Kola	Schisandra
Cat's Claw	Greater Plantain	Shiitake Mushroom
Catuaba	Guazuma	Suma Root
Celandine	Heal-All	Tree Of Life
Chamber Bitter	Holy Basil	Vervain
Chamomile	Indigo	Violet
Chanca Piedra	Jasmine	Winged Treebine
Coleus	Jiaogulan	Wormwood
Coptis	Kamala	Yarrow
Dandelion	Karandas	Yerba Buena
Dang Shen	Lavender	Yerba Buena
Dang Shen	Lavender	Ylang-Ylang
Devil's Claw	Maca Root	Zedoary
Dong Quai	Maitake Mushroom	

That's 74 medicinal plants that can be found as supplements. Bear in mind that they may go by other names and I'll give you a heads up for Red Sorrel: it is sold as Hibiscus Tea and supplements are also available.

17. SOURCES OF KNOWN ANTICANCER PHYTONUTRIENTS
The precious chapter is a review of many phytonutrients that have numerous studies demonstrating anticancer properties and their top plant sources. Some are rich sources of phytonutrients like OLIVES, CAPERS, CACAO, and GREEN TEA no name a few.

CONCLUSION
These lists are far from complete which is surprising because there are already so many plants with amazing anticancer and

immunostimulant properties. And despite the fact that there are many plants that will be very difficult to find in any form there are 147 fruits, vegetables and culinary spices many of which you will be able to find at your local grocery store or order online and another 74 medicinal herbs some that will be on the shelves of your local pharmacy or can be ordered online.

You will notice that many different species of a specific genus of plants are in these lists which means that very likely most if not all of the members of the genus have similar properties. Some examples include: Annona, Morus, Euphorbia, Artocarpus, and Ocimum to name just a few. And when we examine the actual active phytonutrients suspected of having the specific health benefits in these plants we find that they are found throughout the genus. That means that any species in such a genus, even ones not listed here, have the same power. All citrus are loaded with Limonoids, a group of compounds responsible for much of their anticancer power and the Limonoids remain in the blood longer than most other anticancer phytonutrients as well. Many active compounds in the anticancer plants can be found in unrelated plants and they too will have the same anticancer power. Since Quercitin, which has many studies showing it to have anticancer power, found in Mamey and several others in the list, will have anticancer power in any plant that has it, this includes: Apples and Cherries plus Onions are loaded with it. Barley is another grain that contains forms of the Beta-Glucans, found in highest concentrations in most of the edible mushrooms and Oats, that have numerous clinical studies demonstrating that they have measurable, undeniable anticancer and immunostimulant effects and they are present in HUGE quantities in Oats and mushrooms.

Quercitin, beta-Carotene, and Lycopene have all been linked to having either direct anticancer power or definitely the ability to help prevent cancer, and they are all powerful antioxidants and this is why the lists of foods high in antioxidants are so important. Yes, they are most effective in reducing oxidative stress in all cells in the human body which in turn helps curb premature aging and declining organ function and therefore improves overall health and vitality, which is all very desirable, but since many have already have studies proving they have direct anticancer or preventative power, then those foods high in antioxidants, that are not in the Anticancer Plants List, could have measurable anticancer powers as well and they should all be on the top of your list as effective replacements for low quality, low antioxidant, low nutritional value foods.

ABOUT TOXICITY

It is impossible to give a "Short list" of the most effective plants from any of these lists because everyone is different and some plants are not recommended due to various prevailing health conditions of each individual and there is always the possibility that you could be allergic to any of them. Your best approach if you have a chronic condition and are taking medication is to SEEK THE ADVICE OF YOUR DOCTOR BEFORE ADDING HOLISTIC FOODS, SPICES OR MEDICINAL HERBS to your daily intake.

You will get no argument from me that the "in vivo" studies conducted on mice are cruel. But the tests must be done and these animals were bred specifically for these studies (small consolation to the poor mice, I know.) However, they do have surprisingly similar biochemistry, they are more closely related to us than you might care to know and generally speaking what works for them works for us, and what is toxic to them is usually toxic to us. You will also notice that most tests of specific cancers on mice are centered around a relatively limited selection of cell lines like HepG2 hepatocarcinoma. The reason for this is that these cancers can either be transplanted into them or even a few malignant cells can be injected into them, and they will success-fully graft into the mice and grow and ultimately kill them (terrible, I know) and this makes these particular cell lines easy to test in the mice and of great significance because the tests are being done on HUMAN cancers, not always mouse cancers. Once afflicted by these cell lines, the extracts of the plants are administered to see if there is a positive anticancer effect of the extract. If there is, these studies are of great significance because the very same extract could have the same positive effect for humans afflicted with the same form of cancer. This is the second stage of testing (in vitro, is the first stage) and positive results as they accumulate along with results showing the extract to be non-toxic, can ultimately lead to experimental human trials. That however, takes a mountain of positive results from many preliminary tests and in the meantime, there are many people suffering from these cancers who need the help from these plants RIGHT NOW.

I tried to verify that all plants in the lists have either been proven non-toxic (to the mice, and they use huge doses far above what anyone COULD be subjected to) and if the mice don't suffer or die, then I have included those plants in the lists. However, some had no safety study that I could find. Those that did the study and showed the plant to be toxic were mostly removed from the lists. A few remain mainly to illustrate that even toxic plants have shown great promise in anticancer studies like Periwinkle which has already progressed through human trials and its phytochemicals are now the FDA approved cancer treatment drugs Oncovin (Vincristine) and Velban (Vinblastine.)

Because the safety information is sketchy, I always advise anyone thinking of using holistic herbs to USE CAUTION AND MODERATION and SPEAK TO YOUR DOCTOR as well as the vendor of the product. They are very familiar with their products and can warn you of any side effects and potential allergic or toxicity issues.

And repeat it like a mantra: "MORE is NEVER BETTER when it comes to powerful medicines," and many of these plants are very powerful medicines. When taking herbal supplements try to find the lowest dosage on the market and take one and wait a day or two to make sure you don't have any adverse reaction. Try to stick to taking it once or twice a week at the most for cancer prevention; more if you have cancer AND YOUR DOCTOR HAS AGREED to usage of the plant.

Processed cane sugar and high fructose corn syrup have been shown to INCREASE THE RISK OF CANCER AND TO PROMOTE CANCER GROWTH. Foods with high Glycemic Index scores (high in simple sugars and starches) should be AVOIDED if you have cancer and include the BIG 3 FOOD CAUSES of Type II Diabetes: POTATOES, RICE and CORN (eventually I will add WHEAT and all baked goods to this list and call them the Big 4.) These foods in any preparation method have average GI's equal to or worse than Raw Bee Honey and can AGGRAVATE existing chronic conditions including cancer.

Many plants including edibles, spices as well as holistic herbs are loaded with PHYTOESTROGENS. These are compounds produced by the plant that fit into the estrogen receptors of human cells just like estrogen. Because there are many plants loaded with these compounds such as Soybeans that have shown success in combating female hormonal imbalance issues like menopause, they are very popular in holistic medicine. However, there are many forms of cancer that are "hormone-dependent" which means that if estrogen (or androgen) levels rise, these forms of cancer will THRIVE and phytoestrogens could cause this effect. Therefore it is imperative that you NEVER SELF-DIAGNOSE, NEVER SELF-MEDICATE AND IF YOU THINK YOU HAVE CANCER SEE YOUR DOCTOR AND FOLLOW HIS ADVICE AND PROGRAM OF TREATMENT TO THE LETTER AND INFORM HIM OF ALL CHANGES TO YOUR DIET INCLUDING ALL HERBALS YOU ARE TAKING AND/OR PLAN TO TAKE.

OTHER CONCERNS

Always consult with your doctor concerning any changes to your diet or supplement intake because some cancers THRIVE on certain vitamins, minerals and/or specific foods. Many cancers thrive on foods high in sugars and starches that are easily converted into sugars like potatoes, rice and corn. If you have cancer stick to foods with LOW GLYCEMIC INDEX values (foods good for those with Diabetes.)

THANK YOU AND GOD BLESS AND GOOD LUCK AND ABOVE ALL ELSE: TAKE CARE OF YOURSELF (BECAUSE NO ONE ELSE IS GOING TO DO IT)!

SOURCES OF INFORMATION
Annie's Remedy

WEBSITE: www.anniesremedy.com

A valuable online source of information with well over 300 plants listed in their database which was instrumental in the writing of this book. They also sell high quality Essential Oils.

Dr. Godofredo Stuart, Jr. M.D.

WEBSITE: www.stuartxchange.org

This is one of the largest databases of medicinal plants (800+ plants) on the Internet and a valuable tool without which I would not have been able to write this book.

The FDA and the NIH

U.S. Food and Drug Administration: www.fda.gov
National Institutes for Health: www.nih.gov

Both of these governmental agencies have informative websites. Like all governmental agencies, their websites can be difficult to navigate and much of the material is either too simplified or too complicated to be of much value, but I still recommend that you visit them and take a look around.

"DR. AXE"

WEBSITE: www.draxe.com

Josh Axe has an extensive website which I have used as a primary base source of most of the information on the essential nutrients and includes excellent explanations of the health benefits of each one, the nasty results of chronic deficiency for each one, and a list of foods that contain them. The website covers a lot of ground too, not just the "ABC's" (the vitamins and minerals) but also many other health food items and unbiased reports on many supplements like Lycopene, Milk Thistle, and fad products like Creatine, etc.

The George Mateljan Foundation

WEBSITE: www.whfoods.org

This is one of the best reference websites that covers many minerals in excellent detail that most other websites do not. They include a lot of good information on the function of most of the nutrients in the body as well, some of which I could only find at this website and I could never have written this book without their vast collection of nutritional information. They include a lot of additional and useful information about the individual natural whole foods including recipes and weekly diet plans. Check it out.

Wikipedia

WEBSITE: www.wikipedia.org

Wikipedia is an enormous encyclopedia and while some entries on the subject of nutrients are rather limited and also include a lot of talk about the molecular structures and methods of synthesis, it is still one of the best online resources that covers all subjects and each page does include the references which you

113

can pursue as well. Whenever they ask for a few dollars, please give, so we can keep this vast repository of information free and unencumbered by advertising.

"SUPERFOODLY"

WEBSITE ADDRESS: www.superfoodly.com

This site covers a lot of ground and lists the ORAC – Oxygen Radical Absorption Capacity – scores for hundreds of different foods, mostly natural whole foods. I highly recommend this website as a way to "shop for" new antioxidant-rich foods to add to your own natural whole foods diet.

NUTRITION DATA at SELF.COM

WEBSITE: http://nutritiondata.self.com

This is one of the largest repositories of detailed nutrient analyses of a wide range of foods, both packaged as well as natural whole foods, imaginable. The original source of the data is the FDA website, but this website has it in a far better format. Unfortunately, they do not include Molybdenum and Iodine (both covered at the George Mateljan Foundation's website) but the total information provided for each food is still very useful.

"WEB MD"

WEBSITE ADDRESS: www.webmd.com

Aside from having an extensive collection of articles on the nutrients, WebMD also includes many articles on prevention and treatment for just about every ailment as well.

SOURCES OF DIETARY/HERBAL SUPPLEMENTS

GARDEN of LIFE – www.gardenoflife.com – This company makes a whole line of supplements based on natural extract sources of very high quality; many of their products have no competition that I could find: no other natural extract product of the same nutrient(s) on the market, just synthetics. Some of their products are never exposed to temperatures above 115°F which would destroy many nutrients during manufacture. The products are not inexpensive but they are definitely the very best that I could find.

JARROW FORMULAS – www.jarrow.com – This is another manufacturer of very high quality dietary supplements.

NOW FOODS – www.nowfoods.com – An excellent high quality dietary supplement manufacturer.

PURITANS PRIDE – www.puritanspride.com – This vendor also carries many different natural whole food products and supplements as well as their own name brand items.

SWANSON VITAMINS – www.swansonvitamins.com – While they do carry many other brands, this company makes a lot of holistic herbal supplements, many of which can't be found anywhere else.

VITACOST – www.vitacost.com – This is a large online dietary supplement and natural foods vendor. They carry hundreds of brands and also manufacture some very high quality products under their own brand name labels.

APPENDIX B – GLOSSARY OF TERMS

143B cell line – Human osteosarcoma; a form of Bone cancer.

26-M3.1 cell line – A form of lung cancer.

4T1 cell line – A form of breast cancer.

5-FU - 5-Fluorouracil, a standard chemotherapy drug.

A-172 cell line – A form of brain cancer.

A2780 cell line – A form of ovarian cancer.

A375 cell line – A form of melanoma.

A431 cell line – A form of skin cancer.

A498 cell line - Renal cell carcinoma, a form of kidney cancer.

A549 cell line – Human non-small cell lung carcinoma,; a form of lung cancer.

ACF – Aberrant Crypt Foci; a form of colon cancer.

Adenocarcinoma – Forms of cancer that affect organs with mucus membranes.

AGS cell line – Human gastric carcinoma, a form of stomach cancer.

AGZY83-a cell line – A form of lung cancer.

Alcohol – Any organic molecule with a HYDROXYL GROUP attached to any carbon atom in the skeleton is an alcohol.

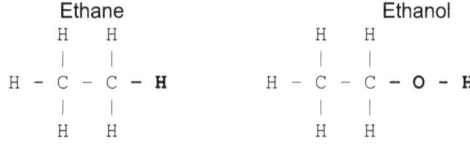

Alkaloid – Any organic compound containing a Nitrogen atom usually within the carbon atom skeleton.

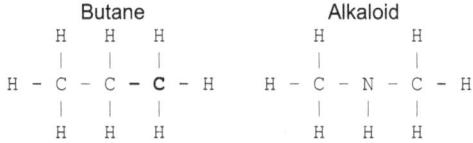

AM-3 cell line – A form of breast cancer.

AMN-3 cell line – A form of breast cancer.

AMPK – Activated Protein Kinase, one of the key molecular pathways by which cancer cells can be selectively targeted and killed.

Antiangiogenesis – Inhibits the formation of new blood vessels, this can severely slow a growing tumor.

Anticancer – Has some capacity to combat cancer.

Anticarcinogenic – Prevents cancer.

Anticlastogenic – Prevents clastogenesis.

Antimetastatic – Prevents metastasis of cancers.

Antimitotic – Prevents cell division (no new cells can be created.)

Antimutagenic – Prevents genetic (DNA) damage in cells.

Antineoplastic – Prevents the creation of new cancerous tissue formation (i.e. tumors.)

Antiosteoclastogenic – Prevents the formation of certain forms of bone cancer.

Antiproliferative – Slows the growth/spread of cancer.

Antithrombotic – Prevents Thrombosis; formation of blood clots in the blood vessels.

Anti-tumor – Has the ability to slow or halt the growth of, or reduce the size of cancerous tumors.

Apoptosis – Cell death caused by a chemically triggered action.

Ascitic tumor – A non-solid tumor.

Autophagic – Pertains to biting or eating oneself; autophagia in cells
means the cells literally consume themselves and die.

B16 cell line – A form of rodent melanoma.

B16F10 cell line – A form of rodent melanoma.

Bcap-37 cell line – A form of breast cancer.

Bcl-2 – A protein that may be a key to defeating cancer cells.

BEL7402 cell line – A form of liver cancer.

Beta-Glucans – A class of small polysaccharides that have been shown in
numerous stiduies to have immunostimulant and anticancer powers.

Benzyl Group – Also called "Phenyl group" or "Aromatic Ring" or "Aryl
group." Molecular structure based on Benzene, a ring of six carbon
atoms:

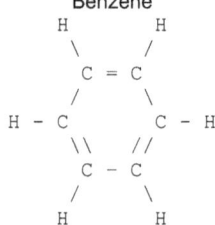

However, the bonds between the six carbon atoms do not actually
alternate single bond, then double bond. All of the bonds between
these atoms are the same length meaning that the bonds constantly
shift locations. This makes the ring both sturdy and uniform in shape
which has had a dramatic effect on all chemistry of all life on Earth.

BGC-823 cell line – A form of stomach cancer

BPH – Benign Prostate Hyperplasia, a form of prostate cancer.

C6 cell line – A form of rodent brain tumor cell.

CaCo-2 cell line – A form of colon cancer.

Calu cell line – A form of lung cancer

Caov-3 cell line - Human ovarian carcinoma.

Capan-1 cell line – A form of pancreatic cancer.

Carcinogen – Causes cancer, usually a chemical.

Carcinogenesis – The beginning of cancer.

Carcinoma – A term for cancer.

CaSki cell line – A form of cervical cancer

CCRF-CEM cell line – A form of leukemia.

CCRF-HSB-2 cell line – Human T-cell leukemia.

CDK – Cyclin-Dependent Kinase; inhibiting CDK can help slow the growth
of cancer especially aggressive tumors.

CEM cell line – A form of leukemia.

CEM-ADR5000 cell line – A drug resistant form of CEM leukemia.

Chalcanoid – Major subcategory of Phenolics, similar in structure to
STILBENOIDS.

Chemoprotective – Prevents damage to DNA in cells caused by chemical
toxins.

Cholesterol – Triterpenoid; Cholesterol is in all animal cell membranes
and is what makes them elastic. The more they need to change
shape, the more cholesterol is incorporated into the cell membranes

(i.e. muscle and skin cells.) The liver manufactures Cholesterol from similar molecules (See PHYTOSTEROLS) found in plants and bundles the cholesterol molecule with one fat (Lipid) molecule and one protein molecule and sends them out into the blood for all cells and tissues to absorb and use. This gives rise to the terms LDL – Low Density Lipoprotein and HDL – High Density Lipoprotein for the packets that the liver makes and sends out into the blood.

Clastogenesis – Formation of breakages. In cancer refers to breakages in DNA that lead to mutated cells that could turn cancerous.

CNE cell line – A form of nasopharyngeal carcinoma; cancer of the mucus membranes of the sinus cavity and throat.

Colo-205 cell line – A form of colon cancer.

Colo-320 cell line – A form of colon cancer.

COR-L23 cell line – Human caucasian large cell lung carcinoma; a form of lung cancer.

Coumarins – Large class of phenolics found in many plants that are mildly toxic to humans in excessive amounts.

COX – Cyclooxygenase proteins, involved in the inflammatory response in tissues, many diseases including cancer depend on COX to do their damage, COX inhibitors are well known for their anti-inflamatory and anticancer power.

Cucurbitacins – Class of Triterpenoids found in abundance in the Cucurbit family. Many of these have been shown to have significant anticancer activity.

Cucurbit – Plants related to Cucumbers and there are many of them. Members feature compounds called Cucurbitacins which have shown a wide range of health benefits including anticancer properties.

CXCR4 – Chemokine Receptor type 4; is an experimental drug target involved in many disease states including 23 types of cancer and several immunodeficiency disorders.

Cytokines – Chemicals produced by the cells that either directly function to provide immunity or call the immune system into action at their location.

Cytoprotective – Protects healthy cells from damage.

Cytotoxic (cytotoxicity) – Poisonous to living cells.

DBMA – 7,12-Dimethylbenzeneanthracene; a well known cancer causing chemical used in live animal cancer studies.

DEN – Diethyl nitrosamine, a known toxin that causes liver damage and liver cancer.

Depurative – Purifies the body or a specific organ or system such as the blood.

Diaphoresis (Diaphoretic) – Promotes the removal of water and toxins through the sweat glands.

Dietary Fiber – A major class of substances found in all edible plants that are by definition "undigestible" in that they do not provide direct nutritional content of any kind. Dietary Fiber, as opposed to "Crude Fiber" is mostly water-soluble and has been shown in myriad studies to improve intestinal health, block Cholesterol absorption and to reduce the risk of colon cancer.

Diterpenoid – Major Category of Phytonutrients based on a skeleton of 20 Carbon atoms (2 Terpene units.)

Diuresis (Diuretic) – Promotes the kidneys to remove water and toxins from the blood.

DAL – Dalton's Ascites Lymphoma, a form of lymphatic cancer.

DLD-1 cell line – A form of colorectal cancer.

DOX – Doxirubicin, a chemical used in chemotherapy.

DU-145 cell line – A form of prostate cancer.

EAC – Ehrlich Ascites Carcinoma, a form of lymphatic cancer.

EBV-EA – Epstein-Barr Virus Early Antigen. Produced by some forms of cancer, inhibition of it can slow the progression of these cancers.

Eca-109 cell line – A form of cancer of the esophagus

EGCG – Epigallocatechin-3-gallate (See Page 96)

EL-4 cell line – A form of thymus cancer in mice

Endometrial – Of or pertaining to the surface lining of an organ, in cancer refers to a class of common cancers of many different organs.

Epidermal – Of or pertaining to the skin.

Erythrocyte – Red blood cell.

FAS – Fatty Acid Synthase, a compound that is strongly created by prostate cancer cells; inhibiting it may inhibit the cancer.

Fatty Acids – A fat with an ORGANIC ACID group attached to it becomes a Fatty Acid. See MONOUNSATURATED FATTY ACID, POLYUNSATURATED FATTY ACID, SATURATED FATTY ACID.

FEK4 cell line – A form of skin cancer.

Flavan-3-ol – Subcategory of the ISOFLAVONOIDS.

Flavonoid – Major Subcategory of Phenolic phytonutrients that includes: ISOFLAVONOIDS. Aurones, and ANTHOCYANIDINS

GBM8401 cell line – A form of brain cancer

Genoprotective – Protects cells from genetic mutation or DNA damage

Genotoxic (Genotoxicity) – Causes genetic damage to living cells.

Glucosinolates – Large category of organic compounds found in most plants that contain sulfur atoms. Many are powerful antioxidants and others have been shown to have various health benefits ranging from lowering cholesterol to actively fighting cancer. Subcategories are: Isothiocyanate Precursors, Organosulfides, Aglycones, Indoles.

Glycosides – Compounds with a specific type of bond to a sugar molecule, and it must be bonded to non-sugar compound.

H1299 cell line – A form of lung cancer.

HA22T cell line – Human hepatocellular carcinoma, a form of liver cancer.

HaCaT cell line – A form of skin cancer

HBL-100 cell line – A form of breast cancer.

HCT-8 cell ine – A form of colorectal cancer.

HCT15 cell line – A form of colon cancer.

HCT116 cell line – A form of colon cancer

HeLa cell line – A form of human cervical cancer.

Hemato- – Of or pertaining to the blood.

Hematological – Pertaining to the blood.

Hematopoeitic – Pertaining to the formation of red blood cells

HEP2 cell line – Human larynx carcinoma, a form of throat cancer.

Hep3B cell line – A form of liver cancer.

Hepato- – Of or pertaining to the Liver.

Hepatocarcinogenesis – The start of liver cancer.

Hepatocarcinoma – Liver cancer.

Hepatocyte – Liver cell.

Hepatoma – Liver cancer.

Hepatoprotective – Protects the liver.

Hepatotoxic – Poisonous to the liver.

HepG2 cell line – A form of liver cancer.

HepG3 cell line – A form of liver cancer.

HIF-1 – HIF-1 is a transcription factor that cancer cells use to adapt to the hypoxic microenvironment caused by rapid tumor growth.

Histoprotective – Protects living tissue from damage.

HL-60 cell line – A form of leukemia.

HNSCC4 cell line – A form of cancer of the head and neck.

HNSCC31 cell line – A form of cancer of the head and neck.

HO-8910 cell line – A form of ovarian cancer.

HONE-1 cell line – A form of cancer of the nose and throat.

HOP-62 cell line – A form of lung cancer.

Hop65 cell line – A form of lung cancer.

HSC-2 cell line – A form of human oral squamous cell cancer.

HSC-3 cell line – A form of human oral squamous cell cancer.

HSG cell line – A form of cancer of the mouth (salivary glands.)

HT-29 cell line – A form of colon cancer.

Hydroxyl Group – The "$-O-H$" pair, an oxygen atom bonded to one hydrogen atom. When it replaces a hydrogen atom anywhere in an organic molecule it turns it into an ALCOHOL.

Immunomodulatory – Assists the immune system.

Immunostimulant – Substance that causes increased production of cells and compounds used by the immune system.

Isoflavonoid – Major Subcategory of Flavonoids with six subcategories: Flavones, Flavonols, Flavanones, Flavanonols, Flavans, Flavan-3-ols.

Hypoglycemic – Lowers blood sugar levels and may help prevent or treat Type II Diabetes.

Hypolipidemic – Lowers blood fat and cholesterol levels.

Hypotensive – Lowers blood pressure.

Hypoxic – Oxygen deprived, believed to be a major cause of cancer.

IGR-OV-1 cell line – A form of ovarian cancer

IL-1β – Interleukin-1beta; produced by the immune system to help fight off invading organisms.

IL-6 – Interleukin-6; produced by the immune system to help fight off invading organisms.

In Vitro – Within a test tube (outside of a living organism.)

In Vivo – Test done within a living organism.

Int-407 cell line – Form of Intestinal cancer.

Intracellular – Within a living cell.

JAR cell line – A form of cancer of the placenta.

Jurkat cell line – A form of leukemia.

K562 cell line – Human caucasian chronic myelogenous leukemia.

KATO III cell line – A form of stomach cancer.

KB cell line – A form of oral cavity cancer.

kDA – KiloDaltons (1000 DA.) 12 Daltons = the mass of one carbon atom.

Ketone Group – An organic molecule with a single oxygen double bonded to one of the carbons in the skeleton is a Ketone.

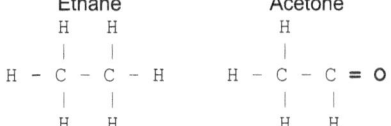

L5178Y cell line – A form of lymphatic cancer.

L-6 cell line – Normal colon cells.

L929 cell line – A form of lung cancer.

LA-7 cells – Normal mammary cells.

Lectins – Proteins that bind to carbohydrates; bacteria and viruses use them to attach to cells as well.

Lignans – Polyphenolics that are also antioxidant phytoestrogens.

LM2 cell line – Mammary adenocarcinoma, a form of breast cancer.

LNCaP cell line – A form of prostate cancer.

LTEP-a-2 cell line – A form of lung cancer.

LU-1 cell line – A form of lung cancer.

Lymphocyte – White blood cell.

M1 cell line – A form of leukemia.

MCF 10A DCIS cell line – A form of breast cancer.

MCF-7 cell line – A hormone-dependent form of breast cancer.

MDA-MB cell line – A form of breast cancer.

MDA-MB-231 cell line – A form of breast cancer.

MDA-MB-435 cell line – A form of breast cancer.

MDA-MB-468 cell line – A form of breast cancer.

Melanogenesis – Formation of Melanoma.

Melanoma – Skin cancer.

Metastasis – Malignant cancer cells colonize other tissues by sending cells through the bloodstream.

MG-63 cell line – Human osteosarcoma; a form of bone cancer.

MGC-803 cell line – A form of stomach cancer.

MHCC97H cell line – A form of liver cancer.

MKN45 cell line – A form of stomach cancer.

MOLT4 cell line – Human acute T-lymphoblastic leukemia.

MMP-9 cell line – A form of breast cancer.

MMK1 – Mitogen-activated Protein Kinase 1; MMK1 is one of the potential targets for cancer therapy that plays a vital role in signal transduction, tumorigenesis, apoptosis and metastasis.

Monophenolic – Phenolic: Contains a single BENZYL GROUP.

Monoterpenoid – Major Category of Phytonutrients based on a skeleton of ten Carbons atoms (Terpene derivatives.)

Monounsaturated Fatty Acid - A fat molecule with one double bond between carbon atoms and that has an ORGANIC ACID group attached. The double bond means that two hydrogen atoms are lost from the chain:

```
        Saturated Fat Section      Monounsaturated Fat Section
        H    H    H    H    H           H                 H    H
        |    |    |    |    |           |                 |    |
   ...- C  - C  - C  - C  - C  -...  ...- C  - C  = C  - C  - C  -...
        |    |    |    |    |           |    |    |    |    |
        H    H    H    H    H           H    H    H    H    H
```

MT-4 cell ine – A form of leukemia.

MUFA – See MONOUNSATURATED FATTY ACID

Murine – Of or pertaining to rodents (mice, etc.)

Mutagen (Mutagenic) – Chemical or Radiation that causes genetic (DNA) damage to living cells.

MV4-11 cell line – A form of leukemia.

Myeloma – A form of cancer of the white blood cells/bone marrow.

NB4 cell line – A form of white blood cell leukemia.

NCI-H69 cell line – A form of lung cancer.

NCI-H187 cell line – Small cell lung cancer.

NCI-H460 cell line – A form of lung cancer.

Neoplasia – Formation of new tissue structures, in cancer, the formation of a new cancer tissue structure (tumor.)

Nephro- – Of or pertaining to the kidneys.

Nephroprotective – Protects the Kidneys.

Neuroprotective – Protects brain cells from damage.

NPC-BM1 cell line – Human nasopharyngeal carcinoma, cancer of the mucus membranes in the sinus cavity and throat.

NSCLC – Non-small cell lung cancer.

Oligosaccharides – Large class of compounds built from simple sugars many of which have shown extraordinary health benefits including immunostimulant and anticancer powers. See beta-Glucans.

Omega-3 Fatty Acid – Polyunsaturated Fatty Acid with a carbon-carbon double bond in position 3 from the end of the molecule, hence the name. Humans cannot make them and they must come from dietary sources: Alpha-Linoleic Acid (ALA) is in plants and Docosahexaenoic Acid (DHA) and Eicosapentaenoic Acid (EPA) are always found together in marine animals ranging from fish to mollusks (i.e. Clams, Scallops, etc) to arthropods (i.e. Crabs, Shrimp, and Lobster.)

Omega-6 Fatty Acid – Polyunsaturated Fatty Acid with a carbon-carbon double bond in position 6 from the end of the molecule, hence the name. The human body cannot synthesize Omega-6's and they are therefore considered to be Essential Nutrients although the amount needed daily is currently being questioned. There are many Omega-6's but gamma-Linoleic Aicd (GLA) and Conjugated Linoleic Acid (CLA) are the most common and found in many plants and unrefined vegetable oils are rich in Omega-6's as are all seeds (i.e. Sunflower Seeds, Sesame Seeds, Flax Seeds, Chia Seeds, etc.) and nuts (i.e. Walnuts, Pecans, etc.) Pomegranate contains a unique form of Linoleic Acid called Punicic Acid as well.

Omega-9 Fatty Acid – Polyunsaturated Fatty Acid with a carbon-carbon double bond in position 9 from the end of the molecule, hence the name. The Omega-9 Fatty Acids can be synthesized in the body, but other Omega-n Fatty Acids are required for this to occur. The most common Omega-9 is Oleic Acid which can be found in many sources of Monunsaturated Fats including Olives and Macadamia nuts.

Organic Acid – **Organic acids differ from mineral aicds (such as Sulfuric** Acid) in the way the Hydrogen that can be freed is attached to the rest of the molecule. Any hydrogen atom can be replaced by an "-O-O-H" group, and the result is an organic acid:

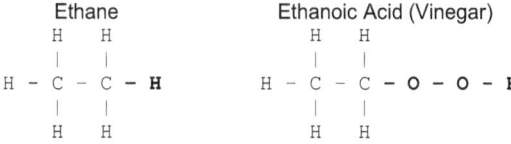

ORAC – Oxygen Radical Absorption Capacity, a measure of the antioxidant potency of a substance.

Osteosarcoma – A form of bone cancer.

OVCAR-3 cell line – Human ovarian cancer

P-gp – P-glycoprotein; its presence in cancer cells is believed to be the major cause of Multidrug Resistance making those cancer cell lines almost immune to most chemotherapy treatments.

P388 cell line – A form of murine leukemia induced in laboratory mice for testing anticancer agents.

PA1 cell line – A form of ovarian cancer.

PACA-2 cell line – A form of human pancreatic cancer.

PANC-1 cell line – A form of Human pancreatic cancer.

Papilloma – Tumor on the surface of an organ and grows outward like a finger.

Papillomagenesis – Formation of papillomas.

PC3 cell line – A form of prostate cancer.

PC3-TxR cell line – A drug resistant form of prostate cancer.

Phenolics – Major Class of phytonutrient compounds. All phenolics have at least one Benzyl group. Major subcategories: FLAVONOIDS, MONOPHENOLICS, POLYPHENOLICS, CHALCANOIDS.

Physalins – Group of molecules specific to plants of the genus Physalis including Cape Gooseberry, Sunberry, etc.

Phytoestrogens – Class of plant compounds that can mimic mammalian estrogen. They have shown efficacy against certain forms of cancer, but could exacerbate others:

Phytosterols – Major subcategory of Terpenoids. The plant sterols are closely related to the animal sterols including Cholesterol. Because of the "-ol" ending in the name they are all alcohols. They also contain carbon rings (though they might not be phenolic in nature) with a specific basic structure of three interlinked benzyl-like rings and a ring of five carbon atoms:

Basic Phytosterol Structure

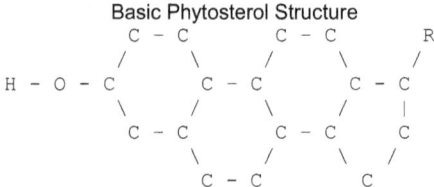

The "R" consists of a branched chain of carbon atoms that varies from one phytosterol to the next and there is also variation in the attached atoms to the carbon atoms shown. You have heard of "one" plant sterol: Vitamin E which is actually eight different forms based on the above basic structure.

PNA – Peanut Agglutination factor; a form of Lectin that binds to D-galactose, a form of sugar.

Polyphenolic – Phenolic: Contains more than one BENZYL GROUP.

Polysaccharides – Complex chains of simple sugars. See beta-Glucans and Oligosaccharides.

Polyunsaturated Fatty Acid – A fat molecule with multiple double bonds between carbon atoms and has an ORGANIC ACID group attached. Each double bond means two hydrogen atoms are lost:

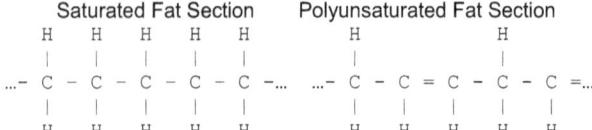

Polysaccharides – Large complex molecular forms of sugar. The beta-Glucans in all edible mushrooms are polysaccharides that have been\

shown to have immunostimulant and anticancer properties. See Oligosaccharides and Page 97 for more details.

PPARγ - Perixome Proliferator-Activated Receptor gamma; a nuclear receptor family transcription factor involved in several types of cancer. This is another molecular key that could lead to effective treatments of cancer.

Pro-apoptotic – Promotes apoptosis; chemically triggered cell death.

PSA – Prostatic Specific Antigen, a key molecular marker in cancer studies.

PUFA – See POLYUNSATURATED FATTY ACID.

Purgative – Strong laxative.

Radioprotective – Protects cells from damage caused by harsh radiation, i.e. short-wave ultraviolet or gamma rays.

Radiotherapy – Use of high energy radiation to kill cancer tissue.

Raji cell line – Burkitt's Lymphoma, a childhood form of lymphatic cancer.

RD cell line – A form of rhabdomyosarcoma; a childhood cancer in which undifferentiated muscle cells turn cancerous.

RDA – Recommended Daily Allowance, published by the Food and Drug Administration.

Renal – Pertaining to the kidneys.

Reno- – Pertaining to the kidneys.

Renoprotective – Protects the kidneys.

RIP – Ribosome-Inactivating Protein; a possible key to defeating cancer.

RKO cell line – A form of colon cancer.

RPMI cell line – A form of plasmacytoma; a mutated white blood cell lodges in soft tissue and grows into a tumor.

S-180 cell line – A form of murine liver cancer.

SaOS-2 cell line – A form of human osteosarcoma, malignant bone cancer.

Saponins – Class of Triterpenoids: Saponins foam when mixed with water and plants rich in them are used to make soap. They are toxic in excess but in small amounts improve digestion and may have other health benefits including anticancer properties.

Sarcoma – A class of cancers.

Saturated Fatty Acid – A fat molecule in which there are no double bonds between any of the carbon atoms in the chains and that has an ORGANIC ACID group attached to it:

```
        Saturated Fat Section        Organic Acid Group Attachment
        H    H    H    H    H             H    H    H
        |    |    |    |    |             |    |    |
   ...- C  - C  - C  - C  - C -...   ...- C  - C  - C  - O  - O  - H
        |    |    |    |    |             |    |    |
        H    H    H    H    H             H    H    H
```

Sesquiterpenoid – Major Category of Phytonutrient based on a skeleton of 15 Carbon atoms (1.5 Terpene units.)

SFA – See SATURATED FATTY ACID

SGC-7901 cell line – Human gastric adenocarcinoma; a form of stomach cancer.

Starch – A large molecule built out of simple sugars attached to each other in long chains. It differs from fats in that most of the oxygen atoms are still in each sugar unit. Starches are much more easily broken down in the digestive tract into a bounty of simple sugars depending on the exact form of the starch.

Stilbenoid – Major subcategory of Phenolic compounds, it is two BENZYL GROUPS with a carbon chain between them with a KETONE GROUP on the chain.

SH-SY5Y cell line – A form of bone marrow cancer.

SiHa cell line – A form of human cervical cancer.

SK-MEL-5 cell line – Human malignant melanoma.

SK-OV-3 cell line – A form of ovarian cancer.

SKBR3 cell line – A form of breast cancer.

SKVLB-1 cell line – A form of ovarian cancer.

SLMT-1 cell line – A form of esophageal squamous carcinoma.

SMMC-7721 cell line – A form of liver cancer.

Splenocyte – Healthy Spleen cells.

SSC-40 cell line – A form of oral cancer.

SW-480 cell line – A form of colon cancer.

T47D cell line – A form of breast cancer.

Tannins – Major subcategory of Phenolic compounds. There are countless tannins in plants and most are huge molecules with up to 400 Carbin atoms in the structure.

TCA8113d – A form of human tongue carcinoma.

TE671 cell line – Cultured cells used to model human medulloblastoma, a form of childhood brain cancer

Terpene – Monoterpenoid: A basic hydrocarbon of 10 Carbon atoms and 16 Hydrogen atoms. The basic structure is used by plants to construct Monoterpenoids, Diterpenoids, Triterpenoids, Tetraterpenoids and Sesquiterpenoids.

Tetraterpenoid – Major Category of Phytonutrient based on a skeleton of 40 Carbon atoms (4 Terpene units.)

Triterpenoid – Major Category of Phytonutrients based on a skeleton of 30 Carbon atoms (3 Terpene units.)

THP-1 cell line – A form of aute monocytic leukemia.

TNF-α – Tumor Necrosis Factor Alpha; a defensive protein created by the immune system that is basically our own natural chemotherapy drug and helping the immune system to produce more of it may hold the key to future successful cancer treatments.

TPA – A known carcinogen that promotes the formation of tumors.

Tumoricidal – Kills tumors.

Tumorigenesis – Creation of tumors.

U-1231 cell line – A form of brain cancer.

U-2 ATCC HTB-96 cell line – A form of bone cancer.

U251 cell line – A form of brain cancer.

U87 cell ine – Human glioblastoma: a form of brain cancer.

U87MG cell line – Human glioblastoma: a form of brain cancer.

U937 cell line – A form of leukemia.

V79 cell line – Rodent lung fibroblast cells cultured for use in studies.

WiDr cell line – A derivative of HT-29 human colon adenocarcinoma

Wil-2NS cell line – A form of lymphatic cancer.

YMB-1 cell line – A form of breast cancer.

.

REFERENCES

[1] Peanuts and peanut butter: www.stuartxchange.org/Mani.html Retrieved 12/5/18

[2] Antioxidants: https://draxe.com/top-10-high-antioxidant-foods/ Retrieved 8/20/18 * http://www.superfoodly.com (ORAC scores) Retrieved 8/29/18

[3] Grapefruit/Pomelo: www.anniesremedy.com/citrus-paradisi-grapefruit.php Retrieved 12/20/18 * www.stuartxchange.org/Suha.html Retrieved 12/5/18

[4] Cabbage: www.stuartxchange.org/Repolyo.html Retrieved 12/5/18

[5] Carrots: www.stuartxchange.org/Karot.html Retrieved 12/5/18

[6] Aerva: www.stuartxchange.org/Taba-ahas.html Retrieved 12/5/18

[7] Cod Liver Oil: https://nutritiondata.self.com/facts/fats-and-oils/628/2 Retrieved 9/12/18

[8] Broccoli: www.stuartxchange.org/ Broccoli.html Retrieved 12/5/18

[9] Grapes, grape seed, and grape juice: https://draxe.com/grapes-nutrition/ Retrieved 9/12/18 * www.anniesremedy.com/vitis-vinifera-grapes.php Retrieved 12/20/18

[10] Garlic: https://www.webmd.com/vitamins/ai/ingredientmono-300/garlic Retrieved 9/18/18 * www.anniesremedy.com/allium-sativum-garlic.php Retrieved 12/20/18 * www.stuartxchange.org/Bawang.html Retrieved 12/5/18

[11] Pumpkin Seeds: https://nutritiondata.self.com/facts/nut-and-seed-products/3141/2 Retrieved 9/12/18 * www.stuartxchange.org/Upo.html Retrieved 12/5/18

[12] Dark chocolate: https://nutritiondata.self.com/facts/sweets/5390/2 Retrieved 9/12/18 * www.stuartxchange.org/Kakaw.html Retrieved 12/5/18

[13] Spirulina: www.anniesremedy.com/arthrospira-platensis-spirulina.php Retrieved 12/20/18

[14] Omega-3 Fatty Acids: https://draxe.com/omega-3-benefits-plus-top-10-omega-3-foods-list/ Retrieved 8/23/18

[15] Oats: https://nutritiondata.self.com/facts/breakfast-cereals/1597/2 Retrieved 9/12/18 * www.anniesremedy.com/avena-sativa-oats.php Retrieved 12/20/18

[16] Green peas: http://whfoods.com/genpage.php?tname=foodspice&dbid=55 Retrieved 3/8/19 * www.stuartxchange.org/Sitsaro.html Retrieved 12/5/18

[17] Omega-6 fatty acids: https://draxe.com/omega-6/ Retrieved 8/20/18

[18] Kelp: Edwards, Rebekah, https://draxe.com/kelp/ Retrieved 4/16/19 * https://nutritiondata.self.com/facts/vegetables-and-vegetable-products/2617/2 Retrieved 3/8/19

[19] Alfalfa: https://www.anniesremedy.com/medicago-sativa-alfalfa.php Retrieved 12/20/18 * https://draxe.com/bean-sprouts Retrieved 4/1/19

[20] Acerola: www.stuartxchange.org/Acerola.html Retrieved 12/5/18

[21] African Sausage Tree: www.stuartxchange.org/AfricanSausageTree.html Retrieved 12/5/18

[22] Agaricus blazei: www.anniesremedy.com/agaricus-blazei-mushroom.php Retrieved 12/20/18

[23] Agave: www.anniesremedy.com/agave-tequilana.php Retrieved 12/20/18 * www.stuartxchange.org/Magey.html 12/5/18

[24] Celery: www.anniesremedy.com/apium-graviolens-celery-seed.php Retrieved 12/20/18 * www.stuartxchange.org/Kintsay.html

[25] Asparagus: http://whfoods.com/genpage.php?tname=foodspice&

dbid=3 Retrieved 3/8/19 * www.stuartxchange.org/ Asparagus.html retrieved 12/5/18

[26] Beets: http://whfoods.com/genpage.php?tname=foodspice&dbid=49 Retrieved 3/8/19

[27] Agrimony: www.anniesremedy.com/agrimonia-eupatoria-agrimony.php Retrieved 12/20/18

[28] Bok Choy: http://whfoods.com/genpage.php?tname=foodspice& dbid=152Retrieved 3/8/19

[29] Allamanda: www.stuartxchange.org/YellowBell.html Retrieved 12/5/18

[30] Button Mushrooms: http://whfoods.com/genpage.php?tname= foodspice&dbid=97 Retrieved 3/8/19

[31] Cantaloupe: http://whfoods.com/genpage.php?tname=foodspice &dbid=17 Retrieved 3/8/19 * www.stuartxchange.org/Melon.html Retrieved 12/5/18

[32] Cashew: http://whfoods.com/genpage.php?tname=foodspice&dbid=98 Retrieved 3/8/19* www.stuartxchange.org/Kasuy.html Retrieved 12/5/18

[33] Aloe: www.stuartxchange.org/Sabila.html Retrieved 12/5/18

[34] Amaranth: www.stuartxchange.org/Kolitis.html Retrieved 12/5/18

[34] Amla: http://whfoods.com/genpage.php?tname=foodspice &dbid=42 Retrieved 3/8/19

[35] Eggplant: http://whfoods.com/genpage.php?tname=foodspice &dbid=22 Retrieved 3/18/19 * www.stuartxchange.org/Talong.html Retrieved 12/5/18

[36] Andrographis: www.stuartxchange.org/ Sinta.html Retrieved 12/5/18 * www.anniesremedy.com/andrographis-paniculata-andrographis.php Retrieved 12/20/18

[37] Coconut: www.anniesremedy.com/cocos-nucifera-coconut-oil.php Retrieved 12/20/18 * www.stuartxchange.org/Niyog2.html Retrieved 12/5/18 * https://draxe.com/coconut-oil-uses/ Retrieved 3/8/19 * https://nutritiondata.self.com/facts/fats-and-oils/508/2 Retrieved 4/4/19

[38] Flax Seed: www.anniesremedy.com/linum-usitatissimum-flax-seed.php Retrieved 12/20/18 * http://whfoods.com/genpage.php ?tname=foodspice&dbid=81 Retrieved 3/8/19

[39] Goji Berry: www.draxe.com/goji/berry/benefits/ Retrieved 3/8/19

[40] Angelica: www.anniesremedy.com/angelica-archangelica-root.php Retrieved 12/20/18

[41] Anise: www.anniesremedy.com/pimpinella-anisum-anise-seed.php Retrieved 12/20/18

[42] Annatto: www.stuartxchange.org/Asuete.html Retrieved 12/5/18

[43] Ant Plant: www.stuartxchange.org/Banghai.html Retrieved 12/5/18

[44] Lettuce: www.stuartxchange.org/Letsugas.html Retrieved 12/5/18

[45] Mango: www.stuartxchange.org/Manga.html Retrieved 12/5/18 * https://nutritiondata.self.com/facts/fruits-and-fruit-juices/1952/2 Retrieved 3/8/19

[46] Olives: http://draxe.com/foods-lower-blood-pressure.html Retrieved 9/10/18 * http://whfoods.com/genpage.php?tname=foodspice &dbid=46 Retrieved 12/5/18

[47] Papaya: http://whfoods.com/genpage.php?tname=foodspice &dbid=47 Retrieved 3/8/19 * www.stuartxchange.org/Papaya.html Retrieved 12/5/18

[48] Aquatic Rotula: www.stuartxchange.org/Takad.html Retrieved 12/5/18

[49] Artillery Plant: www.stuartxchange.org/Alabong.html Retrieved 12/5/18

[50] Okra: https://nutritiondata.self.com/facts/vegetables-and/vegetable-products/2497/2 Retrieved 3/16/19 * https://articles.mercola.com/sites/articles/archive/2016/08/15/health-benefits-of-okra.aspx Retrieved 3/8/19

[51] Onion: www.stuartxchange.org/Sibuyas.html Retrieved 12/5/18 * http://whfoods.com/genpage.php?tname=foodspice&dbid=45 Retrieved 3/8/19

[52] Ashitaba: www.stuartxchange.org/Ashitaba.html Retrieved 12/5/18

[53] Asoka Tree: www.stuartxchange.org/Asoka.html Retrieved 12/5/18

[54] Pineapple: http://whfoods.com/genpage.php?tname=foodspice&dbid=34 Retrieved 3/8/19 * www.stuartxchange.org/Pina.html Retrieved 12/5/18

[55] Astragalus: www.anniesremedy.com/astragalus-membranaceus-root.php Retrieved 12/20/18

[56] Pomegranate: https://www.bbcgoodfood.com/howto/guide/health-benefits-pomegranate Retrieved 3/8/19

[57] Pumpkin: https://nutritiondata.self.com/facts/vegetables-and/vegetable-products/2602/2 Retrieved 3/16/19 * www.stuartxchange.org/Kalabasa.html Retrieved 12/5/18

[58] Bael: www.stuartxchange.org/Bael.html Retrieved 12/5/18

[59] Bamboo Orchid: www.stuartxchange.org/BambooOrchid.html Retrieved 12/5/18

[60] Sesame Seed: http://whfoods.com/genpage.php?tname=foodspice&dbid=84 Retrieved 3/8/19 * www.stuartxchange.org/Linga.html Retrieved 12/5/18

[61] Bandicoot Berry: www.stuartxchange.org/Mali.html Retrieved 12/5/18

[62] Strawberries: http://whfoods.com/genpage.php?tname=foodspice&dbid=32 Retrieved 3/19/19

[63] Barberry: www.anniesremedy.com/berberis-vulgaris-barberry.php Retrieved 12/20/18

[64] Barley Grass: www.anniesremedy.com/hordeum-vulgare-barley-grass.php Retrieved 12/20/18

[65] Tomato: www.stuartxchange.org/Kamatis.html Retrieved 12/5/18 * http://whfoods.com/genpage.php?tname=foodspice&dbid=44 Retrieved 3/19/19

[66] Basil: www.stuartxchange.org/Balanoy.html Retrieved 12/5/18

[67] Bayur: www.stuartxchange.org/Bayog.html Retrieved 12/5/18

[68] Bengal Dayflower: www.stuartxchange.org/BiasBias.html Retrieved 12/5/18

[69] Yams: https://foodfacts.mercola.com/yam.html Retrieved 3/18/19 * https://nutritiondata.self.com/facts/vegetables-and-vegetable-products/2726/2 Retrieved 3/18/19

[70] Bermuda Grass: www.stuartxchange.org/akwadKawaran.html Retrieved 12/5/18

[71] Dietary Fiber: http://www.whfoods.com/genpage.php?tname=nutrient&dbid=50 Retrieved 3/8/19

[72] Betel Pepper: www.stuartxchange.org/Ikmo.html Retrieved 12/5/18

[73] Bignay: www.stuartxchange.org/Bignay.html Retrieved 12/5/18

[74] Beta-Glucan Content: Barry V. McCleary and Anna Draga, "Measurement of β-Glucan in Mushrooms and Mycelial Products" Journal of AOAC International Vol. 99, No. 2. © 2016

[75] Birch: www.anniesremedy.com/betula-alba-birch-bark-leaf.php Retrieved 12/20/18

[76] Bitter Melon: www.stuartxchange.org/Ampalaya.html Retrieved

12/5/18

[77] Black Currant: www.stuartxchange.org/Binayuyo.html Retrieved 12/5/18

[78] Black Myrobalan: www.stuartxchange.org/Komintana.html Retrieved 12/5/18

[79] Boneset: www.anniesremedy.com/eupatorium-perfoliatum-boneset.php Retrieved 12/20/18

[80] Borage: www.anniesremedy.com/borago-officinalis-seed-oil.php Retrieved 12/20/18

[81] Guava: www.stuartxchange.org/Bayabas.html Retrieved 12/5/18 * https://nutritiondata.self.com/facts/fruits-and-fruit-juices/1927/2 Retrieved 3/8/19

[82] Hog Plum: www.stuartxchange.org/Libas.html Retrieved 12/5/18

[83] Bottle Gourd: www.stuartxchange.org/Upo.html Retrieved 12/5/18

[84] Annual Mortality Statistics – Centers for Disease Control: https://www.cdc.gov/nchs/fastats/deaths.htm

[85] Breadfruit: www.stuartxchange.org/Rimas.html Retrieved 12/5/18

[86] Bull's Heart: www.stuartxchange.org/Cherimoya.html Retrieved 12/5/18

[87] Burdock: www.anniesremedy.com/arctium-lappa-burdock-root.php Retrieved 12/20/18

[88] Buri Palm: www.stuartxchange.org/Buri.html Retrieved 12/5/18

[89] Burr Marigold: www.stuartxchange.org/Dadayem.html Retrieved 12/5/18

[90] Bush Mint: www.stuartxchange.org/SuobKabayo.html Retrieved 12/5/18

[91] Caesar Weed: www.stuartxchange.org/Dalupang.html Retrieved 12/5/18

[92] Calabash Tree: www.stuartxchange.org/Dalupang.html Retrieved 12/5/18

[93] Canistel: www.stuartxchange.org/Tiesa.html Retrieved 12/5/18

[94] Canna Lily: www.stuartxchange.org/Espanola.html Retrieved 12/5/18

[95] Cannonball Tree: www.stuartxchange.org/CannonBallTree.html Retrieved 12/5/18

[96] Cape Gooseberry: www.stuartxchange.org/Lobo-lobohan.html Retrieved 12/5/18

[97] Caper Thorn: www.stuartxchange.org/Salimbagat.html Retrieved 12/5/18

[98] Carabao's Teats: www.stuartxchange.org/Hilagak.html Retrieved 12/5/18

[99] Caraway: www.anniesremedy.com/carum-carvi-caraway-seed.php Retrieved 12/20/18

[100] Cardamom: www.anniesremedy.com/elettaria-cardamomum.php Retrieved 12/20/18

[101] Caribbean Slash Pine: www.stuartxchange.org/CubanPine.html Retrieved 12/5/18

[102] Carpetweed: www.stuartxchange.org/Malagoso.html Retrieved 12/5/18

[103] Celandine: www.anniesremedy.com/chelidonium-majus-celandine.php Retrieved 12/20/18

[104] Ceylon Boxwood: www.stuartxchange.org/Malakafe.html Retrieved 12/5/18

[105] Chaff Flower: www.stuartxchange.org/Hangod.html Retrieved 12/5/18

[106] Chaga Mushroom: www.anniesremedy.com/inonotus-obliquus-

chaga-mushroom.php Retrieved 12/20/18

[107] Chamber Bitter: www.stuartxchange.org/Ibaibaan.html Retrieved 12/5/18

[108] Chanca Piedra: www.stuartxchange.org/SampaSampalukan.html Retrieved 12/5/18 * www.anniesremedy.com/phyllanthus-niruri-chanca-piedra.php Retrieved 12/20/18

[109] Chayote: www.stuartxchange.org/Sayote.html Retrieved 12/5/18

[110] Cherimoya: www.stuartxchange.org/Cherimoya.html Retrieved 12/5/18

[111] Chickenweed: www.stuartxchange.org/Sayikan.html Retrieved 12/5/18

[112] Chico Sapodilla: www.stuartxchange.org/Chico.html Retrieved 12/5/18

[113] Chicory: www.anniesremedy.com/cichorium-intybus-chicory-root.php Retrieved 12/20/18

[114] China Rose Hibiscus: www.stuartxchange.org/Gumamela.html Retrieved 12/5/18

[115] Chinese Bell Flower: www.stuartxchange.org/Malbas.html Retrieved 12/5/18

[116] Chinese Burr: www.stuartxchange.org/Kulutkulutan.html Retrieved 12/5/18

[117] Chinese Croton: www.stuartxchange.org/ChineseCroton.html Retrieved 12/5/18

[118]Chinese Juniper: www.stuartxchange.org/Juniper.html Retrieved 12/5/18

[119] Chinese Lantern: www.stuartxchange.org/Putokan.html Retrieved 12/5/18

[120] Chinese Lantern Tree: www.stuartxchange.org/Koron-koron.html Retrieved 12/5/18

[121] Chinese Perfume Plant: www.stuartxchange.org/Sinamomong-sungsong.html Retrieved 12/5/18

[122] Chinese Salacia: www.stuartxchange.org/Matang-ulang.html Retrieved 12/5/18

[123] Chinese Sarsaparilla: www.stuartxchange.org/Sarsaparillang-china.html Retrieved 12/5/18

[124] Chinese Strawberry: www.stuartxchange.org/Cham-poi.html Retrieved 12/5/18

[125] Chinese Wedelia: www.stuartxchange.org/Haganoi-tsina.html Retrieved 12/5/18

[126] Chrysanthemum: www.stuartxchange.org/RosasDeJapon.html Retrieved 12/5/18

[127] Cilantro: www.stuartxchange.org/Kulantro.html Retrieved 12/5/18 * www.anniesremedy.com/coriandrum-sativum-cilantro.php Retrieved 12/20/18

[128] Climbing Fig: www.stuartxchange.org/CreepingFig.html Retrieved 12/5/18

[129] Cloves: www.stuartxchange.org/Duhat.html Retrieved 12/5/18

[130] Club Moss: www.stuartxchange.org/Licopodio.html Retrieved 12/5/18

[131] Cockspur: www.stuartxchange.org/Digkit.html Retrieved 12/5/18

[132] Coleus: www.stuartxchange.org/Oregano.html Retrieved 12/5/18 * www.anniesremedy.com/plectranthus-barbatus-coleus-forskohlii.php Retrieved 12/20/18

[133] Common Cockscomb: www.stuartxchange.org/Kindayohan.html Retrieved 12/5/18

[134] Common Leucas: www.stuartxchange.org/Pansi-pansi.html Retrieved 12/5/18

[135] Confederate Rose: www.stuartxchange.org/Amapola.html Retrieved 12/5/18

[136] Coptis: www.anniesremedy.com/coptis-spp.php Retrieved 12/20/18

[137] Coral Tree: www.stuartxchange.org/Binungang-malapad.html Retrieved 12/5/18

[138] Cordyline: www.stuartxchange.org/TungkodPare.html Retrieved 12/5/18

[139] Creeping Wood Sorrel: www.stuartxchange.org/TaingangDaga.html Retrieved 12/5/18

[140] Crown Flower: www.stuartxchange.org/Kapal-kapal.html Retrieved 12/5/18

[141] Crown of Thorns: www.stuartxchange.org/CoronaDeEspina.html Retrieved 12/5/18

[142] Curry Leaf: www.stuartxchange.org/Karipata.html Retrieved 12/5/18

[143] Custard Apple: www.stuartxchange.org/Atis.html Retrieved 12/5/18

[144] Cut Nut: www.stuartxchange.org/Himbabalod.html Retrieved 12/5/18

[145] Cynometra: www.stuartxchange.org/Oringen.html Retrieved 12/5/18

[146] Dainty Spurs: www.stuartxchange.org/Tagak-tagak.html Retrieved 12/5/18

[147] Dandelion: www.stuartxchange.org/Dandelion.html Retrieved 12/5/18 * www.anniesremedy.com/taraxacum-officinale-dandelion-root.php Retrieved 12/20/18

[148]Desert Purslane: www.stuartxchange.org/Toston.html Retrieved 12/5/18

[149] Devil's Claw: www.anniesremedy.com/harpagophytum-procumbens-devil-claw.php Retrieved 12/20/18

[150] Devil's Tail: www.stuartxchange.org/Kangitngit.html Retrieved 12/5/18

[151] Devil's Tongue: www.stuartxchange.org/Buntot-tigre.html Retrieved 12/5/18

[152] Dong Quai: www.anniesremedy.com/angelica-sinensis-dong-quai.php Retrieved 12/20/18

[153] Dragon Fruit: www.stuartxchange.org/DragonFruit.html Retrieved 12/5/18

[154] Dragon Scales: www.stuartxchange.org/Pagong-pagongan.html Retrieved 12/5/18

[155] Dragon Tail Plant: www.stuartxchange.org/Tabatib.html Retrieved 12/5/18

[156] Drumstick Tree: www.stuartxchange.org/Malunggay.html Retrieved 12/5/18

[157] Duck's Eyes: www.stuartxchange.org/Tagpo.html Retrieved 12/5/18

[158] East Indian Globe Thistle: www.stuartxchange.org/Botobo-tonisan.html Retrieved 12/5/18

[159] Eel Grass: www.stuartxchange.org/Lamon.html Retrieved 12/5/18

[160] Egyptian Grass: www.stuartxchange.org/Damung-balang.html Retrieved 12/5/18

[161] Elderberry: www.stuartxchange.org/Sauko.html Retrieved 12/5/18 * www.anniesremedy.com/sambucus-nigra-elderberry.php Retrieved 12/20/18

[162] Elephant's Foot (E. mollis): www.stuartxchange.org/Malatabako.html Retrieved 12/5/18

[163] Endive: www.stuartxchange.org/Endiba.html Retrieved 12/5/18

[164] Eucalyptus: www.stuartxchange.org/Eucalyptus.html Retrieved 12/5/18 * www.anniesremedy.com/eucalyptus-globulus.php Retrieved 12/20/18

[165] False Daisy: www.stuartxchange.org/Tintatintahan.html Retrieved 12/5/18

[166] False Garlic: www.stuartxchange.org/GarlicVine.html Retrieved 12/5/18

[167] False Heather: www.stuartxchange.org/Kupea.html Retrieved 12/5/18

[168] False Primrose: www.stuartxchange.org/Malapako.html Retrieved 12/5/18

[169] Fennel: www.stuartxchange.org/Haras.html Retrieved 12/5/18 * www.anniesremedy.com/foeniculum-vulgare-fennel-seed.php Retrieved 12/20/18

[170] Fever Bark: www.stuartxchange.org/Dita.html Retrieved 12/5/18

[171] Finger Grass: www.stuartxchange.org/Angangi.html Retrieved 12/5/18

[172] Fish Fern: www.stuartxchange.org/Pakong-alagdan.html Retrieved 12/5/18

[173] Firefly Mangrove: www.stuartxchange.org/Hikau-hikauan.html Retrieved 12/5/18

[174] Five-Leaved Chaste Tree: www.stuartxchange.org/Lagundi.html Retrieved 12/5/18

[175] Flame Vine: www.stuartxchange.org/FlameFlower.html Retrieved 12/5/18

[176] Flamingo Bill: www.stuartxchange.org/Katurai.html Retrieved 12/5/18

[177] Fo-Ti: www.anniesremedy.com/polygonum-multiflorum-fo-ti-root.php Retrieved 12/20/18

[178] Four O'clock: www.stuartxchange.org/AlasCuatro.html Retrieved 12/5/18

[179] Fragrant Glory Bower: www.stuartxchange.org/Pelegrina.html Retrieved 12/5/18

[180] Fragrant Premna: www.stuartxchange.org/Alagaw.html Retrieved 12/5/18

[181] Frangipani: www.stuartxchange.org/Kalachuchi.html Retrieved 12/5/18

[182] Frankincense: www.anniesremedy.com/boswellia-thurifera-boswellia.php Retrieved 12/20/18

[183] Frogfruit: www.stuartxchange.org/Busbusi.html Retrieved 12/5/18

[184] Galangal: www.stuartxchange.org/Dusol.html Retrieved 12/5/18

[185] Galangal Ginger: www.stuartxchange.org/Lankauas.html Retrieved 12/5/18

[186] Gardenia: www.stuartxchange.org/Rosal.html Retrieved 12/5/18

[187] Gerbera Daisy: www.stuartxchange.org/AfricanDaisy.html Retrieved 12/5/18

[188] Ghost Flower: www.stuartxchange.org/Dapong-tubo.html Retrieved 12/5/18

[189] Gin Berry: www.stuartxchange.org/Gingging.html Retrieved 12/5/18

[190] Ginger: www.stuartxchange.org/Luya.html Retrieved 12/5/18 * www.anniesremedy.com/zingiber-officinale-ginger-root.php Retrieved 12/20/18

[191] Glabrous Sarcandra: www.stuartxchange.org/Apot.html Retrieved 12/5/18

[192] Globe Amarathus: www.stuartxchange.org/Botoncillo.html Retrieved 12/5/18

[193] Goat Weed: www.stuartxchange.org/Bulak.html Retrieved 12/5/18
[194] Gold Dust Dracaena: www.stuartxchange.org/SpottedDracaena.html
Retrieved 12/5/18
[195] Golden Eye Grass: www.stuartxchange.org/Taloangi.html Retrieved
12/5/18
[196] Golden Leather Fern: www.stuartxchange.org/Lagolo.html Retrieved
12/5/18
[197] Golden Rod: www.stuartxchange.org/Tantanduk.html Retrieved
12/5/18 * www.anniesremedy.com/solidago-virgaurea-goldenrod.php
Retrieved 12/20/18
[198] Gotu Kola: www.stuartxchange.org/TakipKohol.html Retrieved
12/5/18 * www.anniesremedy.com/centella-asiatica-gotu-kola.php
Retrieved 12/20/18
[199] Governor's Plum: www.stuartxchange.org/Palutan.html Retrieved
12/5/18
[200] Greater Plantain: www.stuartxchange.org/Lanting.html Retrieved
12/5/18 * www.anniesremedy.com/plantago-major-lanceolata-
plantain.php Retrieved 12/20/18
[201] Guazuma: www.stuartxchange.org/Guazuma.html Retrieved 12/5/18
[202] Heal-all: www.anniesremedy.com/prunella-vulgaris-self-heal.php
Retrieved 12/20/18
[203] Heartleaf Hempvine: www.stuartxchange.org/Bikas.html Retrieved
12/5/18
[204] Hen's Eyes: www.stuartxchange.org/CoralBerry.html Retrieved
12/5/18
[205] Holly-leaved Acanthus: www.stuartxchange.org/Diluario.html
Retrieved 12/5/18
[206] Holy Basil: www.stuartxchange.org/Sulasi.html Retrieved 12/5/18 *
www.anniesremedy.com/ocimum-sanctum-holy-basil.php Retrieved
12/20/18
[207] Horsetail: www.stuartxchange.org/Horsetail.html Retrieved 12/5/18
[208] Honeybush: www.anniesremedy.com/cyclopia-honeybush.php
Retrieved 12/20/18
[209] Hummingbird Bush: www.stuartxchange.org/DonManuel.html
Retrieved 12/5/18
[210] Indian Hemp: www.stuartxchange.org/AlasDoce.html Retrieved
12/5/18
[211] Indian Mangrove: www.stuartxchange.org/Api-api.html Retrieved
12/5/18
[212] Indian Marshweed: www.stuartxchange.org/Tara-tara.html Retrieved
12/5/18
[213] Indian Patchouli: www.stuartxchange.org/Kadlum.html Retrieved
12/5/18
[214] Indian Snowberry: www.stuartxchange.org/Matang-hipon.html
Retrieved 12/5/18
[215] Indian Zehneria: www.stuartxchange.org/Melon-daga.html Retrieved
12/5/18
[216] Indigo: www.stuartxchange.org/Tina-tinaan.html Retrieved 12/5/18
[217] Insulin Plant: www.stuartxchange.org/InsulinPlant.html Retrieved
12/5/18
[218] Ironweed: www.stuartxchange.org/AgasMoro.html Retrieved 12/5/18
[219] Ironwood Tree: www.stuartxchange.org/Kolis.html Retrieved 12/5/18
[220] Ivory Mahogany: www.stuartxchange.org/Igiu.html Retrieved 12/5/18
[221] Ivy-rue: www.stuartxchange.org/Kayetana.html Retrieved 12/5/18

[222] Ixora: www.stuartxchange.org/Santan.html Retrieved 12/5/18

[223] Jaboticaba: www.stuartxchange.org/Jaboticaba.html Retrieved 12/5/18

[224] Jackfruit: www.stuartxchange.org/Langka.html Retrieved 12/5/18

[225] Jamaican Cherry: www.stuartxchange.org/Aratiles.html Retrieved 12/5/18

[226] Japanese Alnus: www.stuartxchange.org/Arnus.html Retrieved 12/5/18

[227] Jasmine: www.stuartxchange.org/Jasmin.html Retrieved 12/5/18

[228] Judas Ear: www.stuartxchange.org/Taingan-daga.html Retrieved 12/5/18

[229] Job's Tears: www.stuartxchange.org/Katigbi.html Retrieved 12/5/18

[230] Joe-Pye Weed: www.anniesremedy.com/eupatorium-purpureum-joe-pye-weed.php Retrieved 12/20/18

[231] Joshua Tree: www.anniesremedy.com/yucca-root.php Retrieved 12/20/18

[232] Jujube: www.stuartxchange.org/Mansanitas.html Retrieved 12/5/18

[233] Jute: www.stuartxchange.org/PasauNaBilog.html Retrieved 12/5/18

[234] Kamala: www.stuartxchange.org/Kalpueng.html Retrieved 12/5/18

[235] Karandas: www.stuartxchange.org/Caranda.html Retrieved 12/5/18

[236] Knobweed: www.stuartxchange.org/Botonesan.html Retrieved 12/5/18

[237] Knotweed: www.stuartxchange.org/Subsuban.html Retrieved 12/5/18

[238] Kudzu: www.stuartxchange.org/Baai.html Retrieved 12/5/18

[239] Langsat: www.stuartxchange.org/Lansones.html Retrieved 12/5/18

[240] Laurel Fern: www.stuartxchange.org/PakongParang.html Retrieved 12/5/18

[241] Lavender: www.stuartxchange.org/Lavandula.html Retrieved 12/5/18

[242] Leichhardt Tree: www.stuartxchange.org/Bangkal.html Retrieved 12/5/18

[243] Lemon Grass: www.stuartxchange.org/Tanglad.html Retrieved 12/5/18

[244] Leopard Lily: www.stuartxchange.org/Abaniko.html Retrieved 12/5/18

[245] Licorice: www.stuartxchange.org/Licorice.html Retrieved 12/5/18 * www.anniesremedy.com/glycyrrhiza-glabra-licorice-root.php Retrieved 12/20/18

[246] Lime: www.stuartxchange.org/Dayap.html Retrieved 12/5/18 * www.anniesremedy.com/citrus-aurantifolia-lime-oil.php Retrieved 12/20/18

[247] Lolly Fruit: www.stuartxchange.org/Santol.html Retrieved 12/5/18

[248] Long Pepper: www.stuartxchange.org/Litlit.html Retrieved 12/5/18

[249] Lotus: www.stuartxchange.org/Baino.html Retrieved 12/5/18

[250] Lotus Lily: www.stuartxchange.org/Lauas.html Retrieved 12/5/18

[251] Love Grass: www.stuartxchange.org/Amor-seco.html Retrieved 12/5/18

[252] Lychee: www.stuartxchange.org/Litsiyas.html Retrieved 12/5/18

[253] Madder: www.stuartxchange.org/Mankit.html Retrieved 12/5/18

[254] Maitake Mushroom: www.anniesremedy.com/grifola-frondosa-maitake-mushroom.php Retrieved 12/20/18

[255] Malay Apple: www.stuartxchange.org/Makopa.html Retrieved 12/5/18

[256] Mamey: www.stuartxchange.org/Chico-mamei.html Retrieved 12/5/18

[257] Mangosteen: www.stuartxchange.org/Mangosteen.html Retrieved 12/5/18

[258] Marang: www.stuartxchange.org/Marang.html Retrieved 12/5/18

[259] Marjoram: www.anniesremedy.com/origanum-majorana-marjoram-sweet.php Retrieved 12/20/18
[260] Marsh Fleabane: www.stuartxchange.org/Kalapini.html Retrieved 12/5/18
[261] Marsh Mallow: www.stuartxchange.org/Barulad.html Retrieved 12/5/18
[262] Milk Hedge: www.stuartxchange.org/Bali-bali.html Retrieved 12/5/18
[263] Mimosa: www.stuartxchange.org/Makahiya.html Retrieved 12/5/18
[264] Miracle Fruit: www.stuartxchange.org/MiracleFruit.html Retrieved 12/5/18
[265] Mulberry: www.stuartxchange.org/Morera.html Retrieved 12/5/18
[266] Mullein Nightshade: www.stuartxchange.org/Malatalong.html Retrieved 12/5/18
[267] Musk Mallow: www.stuartxchange.org/Kastuli.html Retrieved 12/5/18
[268] Mustard: www.stuartxchange.org/Mustasa.html Retrieved 12/5/18 * www.anniesremedy.com/brassica-nigra-mustard.php Retrieved 12/20/18
[269] Neem: www.stuartxchange.org/Neem.html Retrieved 12/5/18 * www.anniesremedy.com/azadirachta-indica-neem.php Retrieved 12/20/18
[270] Nicker Tree: www.stuartxchange.org/Kalumbibit.html Retrieved 12/5/18
[271] Night Blooming Jessamine: www.stuartxchange.org/DamaDeNoche.html Retrieved 12/5/18
[272] Nipple Fruit: www.stuartxchange.org/Utong.html Retrieved 12/5/18
[273] Noni: www.stuartxchange.org/Apatot.html Retrieved 12/5/18
[274] Norfolk Pine: www.stuartxchange.org/NorfolkPine.html Retrieved 12/5/18
[275] Nut Grass: www.stuartxchange.org/Mutha.html Retrieved 12/5/18
[276] Orange Climber: www.stuartxchange.org/Dawag.html Retrieved 12/5/18
[277] Orchid Tree: www.stuartxchange.org/OrchidTree.html Retrieved 12/5/18
[278] Oregano: www.anniesremedy.com/origanum-vulgare-oregano.php Retrieved 12/20/18
[279] Otaheite Gooseberry: www.stuartxchange.org/Iba.html Retrieved 12/5/18
[280] Parsley: www.stuartxchange.org/Parsley.html Retrieved 12/5/18 * www.anniesremedy.com/petroselinum-crispum-parsley.php Retrieved 12/20/18
[281] Passion Fruit: www.stuartxchange.org/Pasyonaryo.html Retrieved 12/5/18
[282] Pastureweed: www.stuartxchange.org/Dayang.html Retrieved 12/5/18
[283] Patchouli: www.stuartxchange.org/Kabling.html Retrieved 12/5/18
[284] Pau D'arco: www.anniesremedy.com/tabebuia-spp-pau-d-arco.php Retrieved 12/20/18
[285] Peacock Moss: www.stuartxchange.org/PeacockMoss.html Retrieved 12/5/18
[286] Pearl Grass: www.stuartxchange.org/MalaUlasiman.html Retrieved 12/5/18
[287] Periwinkle: www.stuartxchange.org/Tsitsirika.html Retrieved 12/5/18
[288] Philippine Almond: www.stuartxchange.org/Kalamansanai.html Retrieved 12/5/18

[289] Philippine Cedar: www.stuartxchange.org/Kalantas.html Retrieved 12/5/18

[290] Pigeon Pea: www.stuartxchange.org/Kadios.html Retrieved 12/5/18

[291] Pili Nut: www.stuartxchange.org/Pili.html Retrieved 12/5/18

[292] Pinecone Ginger: www.stuartxchange.org/Luiang-usiu.html Retrieved 12/5/18

[293] Pink Wampee: www.stuartxchange.org/Buringit.html Retrieved 12/5/18

[294] Polyanthus Lily: www.stuartxchange.org/Azucena.html Retrieved 12/5/18

[295] Popping Pod: www.stuartxchange.org/Ruellia.html Retrieved 12/5/18

[296] Portia Tree: www.stuartxchange.org/Banago.html Retrieved 12/5/18

[297] Potato Bush: www.stuartxchange.org/Malatinta.html Retrieved 12/5/18

[298] Pouzolzs Bush: www.stuartxchange.org/Tuia.html Retrieved 12/5/18

[299] Prickly Ash: www.stuartxchange.org/Kangai.html Retrieved 12/5/18

[300] Prickly Poppy: www.stuartxchange.org/Kachumba.html Retrieved 12/5/18

[301] Purple Tephrosia: www.stuartxchange.org/Balatong-pula.html Retrieved 12/5/18

[302] Purslane: www.stuartxchange.org/Gulasiman.html Retrieved 12/5/18

[303] Puzzlenut Tree: www.stuartxchange.org/Piyagaw.html Retrieved 12/5/18

[304] Radish: www.stuartxchange.org/Labanos.html Retrieved 12/5/18

[305] Rambutan: www.stuartxchange.org/Rambutan.html Retrieved 12/5/18

[306] Red Clover: www.anniesremedy.com/trifolium-pratense-red-clover.php Retrieved 12/20/18

[307] Red Cotton: www.stuartxchange.org/Bulak-damo.html Retrieved 12/5/18

[308] Red Ginger: www.stuartxchange.org/RedGinger.html Retrieved 12/5/18

[309] Red Sorrel: www.stuartxchange.org/Roselle.html Retrieved 12/5/18

[310] Red Tree Vine: www.stuartxchange.org/Abang-Abang.html Retrieved 12/5/18

[311] Reishi Mushroom: www.anniesremedy.com/ganoderma-lucidum-reishi-mushroom.php Retrieved 12/20/18

[312] Resurrection Plant: www.stuartxchange.org/Katakataka.html Retrieved 12/5/18

[313] Ribbon Plant: www.stuartxchange.org/SpiderPlant.html Retrieved 12/5/18

[314] Rooibos: www.anniesremedy.com/aspalathus-linearis-rooibos.php Retrieved 12/20/18

[315] Rose: www.stuartxchange.org/Rose.html Retrieved 12/5/18 * www.anniesremedy.com/rosa-spp-rose.php Retrieved 12/20/18

[316] Rose Leadwort: www.stuartxchange.org/Laurel.html Retrieved 12/5/18

[317] Rosemary: www.stuartxchange.org/Romero.html Retrieved 12/5/18 * www.anniesremedy.com/rosmarinus-officinalis-rosemary.php Retrieved 12/20/18

[318] Royal Poinciana: www.stuartxchange.org/FireTree.html Retrieved 12/5/18

[319] Rubber Plant: www.stuartxchange.org/Balete.html Retrieved 12/5/18

[320] Sacred Fig: www.stuartxchange.org/BoTree.html Retrieved 12/5/18

[321] Safflower: www.stuartxchange.org/Kasubha.html Retrieved 12/5/18
[322] Sage: www.stuartxchange.org/Sage.html Retrieved 12/5/18 *
www.anniesremedy.com/salvia-officinalis-sage.php Retrieved
12/20/18
[323] Sandpaper Tree: www.stuartxchange.org/Kalios.html Retrieved
12/5/18
[324] Sappan Wood: www.stuartxchange.org/Sapan.html Retrieved
12/5/18
[325] Screw Pine: www.stuartxchange.org/Pandan.html Retrieved 12/5/18
[326] Sea Rosemallow: www.stuartxchange.org/Malabago.html Retrieved
12/5/18
[327] Seaside Plum: www.stuartxchange.org/Buol.html Retrieved 12/5/18
[328] Septic Fig: www.stuartxchange.org/Hauili.html Retrieved 12/5/18
[329] Shaggy Buttonweed: www.stuartxchange.org/Landrina.html
Retrieved 12/5/18
[330] Shallot: www.stuartxchange.org/SibuyasTagalog.html Retrieved
12/5/18
[331] Shiny Bush: www.stuartxchange.org/Pansit.html Retrieved 12/5/18
[332] Beta-Glucans: https://www.fxmedicine.com.au/blog-post/beta-
glucans-medicinal-actives-mushrooms
[333] Shoofly: www.stuartxchange.org/Puto.html Retrieved 12/5/18
[334] Sicklepod: www.stuartxchange.org/Katanda.html Retrieved 12/5/18
[335] Singapore Rhododendron: www.stuartxchange.org/Malatungaw.html
Retrieved 12/5/18
[336] Slender Carpetweed: www.stuartxchange.org/Sarsalida.html
Retrieved 12/5/18
[337] Smartweed: www.stuartxchange.org/Buding.html Retrieved 12/5/18
[338] Snake Gourd: www.stuartxchange.org/Melon-melonan.html Retrieved
12/5/18
[339] Snake Needle Grass: www.stuartxchange.org/UlasimanKalat.html
Retrieved 12/5/18
[340] Snake Weed: www.stuartxchange.org/GatasGatas.html Retrieved
12/5/18
[341] Sneeze Weed: www.stuartxchange.org/Harangan.html Retrieved
12/5/18
[342] Sour Orange: www.anniesremedy.com/citrus-z-aurantium-bitter-
range.php Retrieved 12/20/18[sic]
[343] Soursop: www.stuartxchange.org/Guyabano.html Retrieved 12/5/18
[344] Sow Thistle: www.stuartxchange.org/Gagatang.html Retrieved
12/5/18
[345] Spider Flower: www.stuartxchange.org/SeruWalai.html Retrieved
12/5/18
[346] Spreading Hogweed: www.stuartxchange.org/Paanbalibis.html
Retrieved 12/5/18
[347] St. Paul's Wort: www.stuartxchange.org/Put.html Retrieved 12/5/18
[348] Star Apple: www.stuartxchange.org/Caimito.html Retrieved 12/5/18
[349] Star Fruit: www.stuartxchange.org/Balimbing.html Retrieved 12/5/18
[350] Stinkvine: www.stuartxchange.org/Kantutan.html Retrieved 12/5/18
[351] Suma Root: www.anniesremedy.com/pfaffia-paniculata-suma-
root.php Retrieved 12/20/18
[352] Sunberry: www.stuartxchange.org/UntiUntihan.html Retrieved
12/5/18
[353] Sweet Acacia: www.stuartxchange.org/Aroma.html Retrieved 12/5/18
[354] Sweet Broom: www.stuartxchange.org/Malaanis.html Retrieved

12/5/18

[355] Sweet Violet: www.stuartxchange.org/Violeta.html Retrieved 12/5/18 * www.anniesremedy.com/viola-spp-violet-leaf.php Retrieved 12/20/18

[356] Tailed Maidenhair: www.stuartxchange.org/Alambrillong-gubat.html Retrieved 12/5/18

[357] Taiwan Goniothalamus: www.stuartxchange.org/Amuyon.html Retrieved 12/5/18

[358] Tamarind: www.stuartxchange.org/Sampalok.html Retrieved 12/5/18

[359] Tangle Fern: www.stuartxchange.org/Kilob.html Retrieved 12/5/18

[360] Taro: www.stuartxchange.org/Gabi.html Retrieved 12/5/18

[361] Tea: www.stuartxchange.org/Tsa.html Retrieved 12/5/18 * www.anniesremedy.com/camellia-sinensis-tea.php Retrieved 12/20/18

[362] Three-Leaf Cayratia: www.stuartxchange.org/Kalit-kalit.html Retrieved 12/5/18

[363] Three-Leaved Chaste Tree: www.stuartxchange.org/Lagunding-dagat.html Retrieved 12/5/18

[364] Thryallis: www.stuartxchange.org/Kuisia.html Retrieved 12/5/18

[365] Tick Tree: www.stuartxchange.org/Dikit-dikit.html Retrieved 12/5/18

[366] Tiger's Claw: www.stuartxchange.org/Dapdap.html Retrieved 12/5/18

[367] Torch Ginger: www.stuartxchange.org/TorchGinger.html Retrieved 12/5/18

[368] Touch-Me-Not: www.stuartxchange.org/Kamantigi.html Retrieved 12/5/18

[369] Tree Bean: www.stuartxchange.org/Kupang.html Retrieved 12/5/18

[370] Tree of India: www.stuartxchange.org/IndianTree.html Retrieved 12/5/18

[371] Tree of Life: www.stuartxchange.org/ArborVitae.html Retrieved 12/5/18 * www.anniesremedy.com/thuja-occidentalis-oil.php Retrieved 12/20/18

[372] Tridax Daisy: www.stuartxchange.org/CoatButtons.html Retrieved 12/5/18

[373] Tropical Chickweed: www.stuartxchange.org/Bakalanga.html Retrieved 12/5/18

[374] Turmeric: www.stuartxchange.org/Dilaw.html Retrieved 12/5/18 * www.anniesremedy.com/curcuma-longa-turneric.php Retrieved 12/20/18

[375] Turpeth Tree: www.stuartxchange.org/Bangbangau.html Retrieved 12/5/18

[376] Vanilla: https://draxe.com/vanilla-oil/ Retreived 6/30/19

[377] Velvet Leaf: www.stuartxchange.org/Sansau.html Retrieved 12/5/18

[378] Vervain: www.stuartxchange.org/Verbena.html Retrieved 12/5/18

[379] Wampee: www.stuartxchange.org/Wampi.html Retrieved 12/5/18

[380] Wandering Zebrina: www.stuartxchange.org/Sebrina.html Retrieved 12/5/18

[381] Water Cress: www.stuartxchange.org/Kangkong-kalabau.html Retrieved 12/5/18

[382] Water Hyacinth: www.stuartxchange.org/WaterHyacinth.html Retrieved 12/5/18

[383] Water Hyssop: www.stuartxchange.org/Ulasimang-aso.html Retrieved 12/5/18

[384] Water Pennywort: www.stuartxchange.org/Kanapa.html Retrieved 12/5/18

[385] Water Plantain: www.stuartxchange.org/Kalabua.html Retrieved 12/5/18

[386] Water Spinach: www.stuartxchange.org/Kangkong.html Retrieved 12/5/18

[387] White Berry Bush: www.stuartxchange.org/Botolan.html Retrieved 12/5/18

[388] White Flowered Mangrove: www.stuartxchange.org/Kulasi.html Retrieved 12/5/18

[389] Wild Hops: www.stuartxchange.org/Panapanarahan.html Retrieved 12/5/18

[390] Wild Raspberry: www.stuartxchange.org/Sapinit.html Retrieved 12/5/18

[391] Wild Tea: www.stuartxchange.org/Tsaang.html Retrieved 12/5/18

[392] Winged Treebine: www.stuartxchange.org/Sugpon-sugpon.html Retrieved 12/5/18

[393] Winter Aster: www.stuartxchange.org/Manzanilla.html Retrieved 12/5/18

[394] Wire Grass: www.stuartxchange.org/Paragis.html Retrieved 12/5/18

[395] Wire Bush: www.stuartxchange.org/Bankalanan.html Retrieved 12/5/18

[396] Wormwood: www.stuartxchange.org/Damong.html Retrieved 12/5/18

[397] Yard Long Bean: www.stuartxchange.org/Sitaw.html Retrieved 12/5/18

[398] Yarrow: www.stuartxchange.org/Milfoil.html Retrieved 12/5/18 * www.anniesremedy.com/achillea-millefolium-yarrow.php Retrieved 12/20/18

[399] Yellow Eyed Grass: www.stuartxchange.org/Mala-bawang.html Retrieved 12/5/18

[400] Yellow Sanchezia: www.stuartxchange.org/Sanchezia.html Retrieved 12/5/18

[401] Yerba Buena: www.stuartxchange.org/YerbaBuena.html Retrieved 12/5/18

[402] Ylang-ylang: www.stuartxchange.org/IlangIlang.html Retrieved 12/5/18

[403] Zedoary: www.stuartxchange.org/LuyaLuyahan.html Retrieved 12/5/18

[404] Açai: www.anniesremedy.com/euterpe-oleracea-acai-berry.php Retrieved 12/20/18

[405] Arrowroot: www.stuartxchange.org/Araro.html Retrieved 12/5/18

[406] Beach Morning Glory: www.stuartxchange.org/Bagasua.html Retrieved 12/5/18

[407] Indian Heliotrope: www.stuartxchange.org/TrompangElepante.html Retrieved 12/5/18

[408] Scarlet Bush: www.stuartxchange.org/DonManuel.html Retrieved 12/5/18

[409] Rhodiola: www.anniesremedy.com/rhodiola-rosea-rhodiola.php Retrieved 12/20/18

[410] Quassia: www.stuartxchange.org/Manunggal.html Retrieved 12/5/18

[411] Avocado: www.stuartxchange.org/Abukado.html Retrieved 12/5/18

[412] Lilac Tassleflower: www.stuartxchange.org/Tagulinaw.html Retrieved 12/5/18

[413] Java Brucea: www.stuartxchange.org/Balaniog.html Retrieved 12/5/18

[414] Tropical Almond: www.stuartxchange.org/Talisay.html Retrieved 12/5/18

[415] Henna: www.stuartxchange.org/Sinamomo.html Retrieved 12/5/18

[416] Velvet Bean: www.stuartxchange.org/Nipai.html Retrieved 12/5/18

[417] Circassian Bean: www.stuartxchange.org/SagaHutan.html Retrieved 12/5/18

[418] Kalanchoe: www.stuartxchange.org/Siempreviva.html Retrieved 12/5/18

[419] Bishop's Weed: www.stuartxchange.org/Damoro.html Retrieved 12/5/18 * www.anniesremedy.com/trachyspermum-ammi-ajwain-seed.php Retrieved 12/20/18

[420] Bupleurum: www.anniesremedy.com/bupleurum-chinense-bupleurum.php Retrieved 12/20/18

[421] Capers: www.stuartxchange.org/Dauag.html Retrieved 12/5/18

[422] Cat's Claw: www.anniesremedy.com/uncaria-tomentosa-cat-claw.php Retrieved 12/20/18

[423] Catuaba: www.anniesremedy.com/erythroxylum-catuaba.php Retrieved 12/20/18

[424] Chamomile: www.anniesremedy.com/matricaria-recutita-chamomile.php Retrieved 12/20/18

[425] Cut-Leaved Panax: www.stuartxchange.org/Papua.html Retrieved 12/5/18

[426] Dang Shen: www.anniesremedy.com/codonopsis-pilosula-dang-shen.php Retrieved 12/20/18

[427] Dates: www.stuartxchange.org/DatePalm.html Retrieved 12/5/18

[428] Durian: www.stuartxchange.org/Durian.html Retrieved 12/5/18

[429] Dwarf Geometry Tree: www.stuartxchange.org/Bucida.html Retrieved 12/5/18

[430] Echinacea: www.anniesremedy.com/echinacea-augustifolia.php Retrieved 12/20/18

[431] Eleuthero: www.anniesremedy.com/eleutherococcus-senticosus-eleuthero-root.php Retrieved 12/20/18

[432] Electric Daisy: www.stuartxchange.org/Biri.html Retrieved 12/5/18

[433] Epimedium: www.anniesremedy.com/epimedium=grandiflorum.php Retrieved 12/20/18

[434] Evening Primrose: www.anniesremedy.com/oenothera-biennis-evening-primrose-oil.php Retrieved 12/20/18

[435] Ginkgo Biloba: www.stuartxchange.org/Ginkgo.html Retrieved 12/5/18 * www.anniesremedy.com/ginkgo-biloba.php Retrieved 12/20/18

[436] Ginseng: www.anniesremedy.com/panax-ginseng-root.php Retrieved 12/20/18

[437] Goldenseal: www.anniesremedy.com/hydrastis-canadensis-goldenseal.php Retrieved 12/20/18

[438] Heavenly Elixir: www.stuartxchange.org/Makabuhay.html Retrieved 12/5/18

[439] Jiaogulan: www.anniesremedy.com/gynostemma-pentaphyllum-jiaogulan.php Retrieved 12/20/18

[440] Luffa: www.stuartxchange.org/PatolangBilog.html Retrieved 12/5/18

[441] Maca Root: www.anniesremedy.com/lepidium-peruvianum-maca-root.php Retrieved 12/20/18

[442] Oregon Grape Root: www.anniesremedy.com/mahonia-aquifolium-oregon-grape-root.php Retrieved 12/20/18

[443] Porcupine Flower: www.stuartxchange.org/Kolinta.html Retrieved 12/5/18

[444] Portulaca: www.stuartxchange.org/Portulaca.html Retrieved 12/5/18

[445] Prickly Chaff Flower: www.stuartxchange.org/Hangod.html Retrieved 12/5/18

[446] Schisandra: www.anniesremedy.com/schisandra-chinensis.php Retrieved 12/20/18

[447] Sea Buckthorn: www.anniesremedy.com/hippophae-rhamnoides-sea-buckthorn-oil.php Retrieved 12/20/18

[448] Speargrass: www.stuartxchange.org/Kogon.html Retrieved 12/5/18

[449] Sugar cane: www.stuartxchange.org/Tubo.html Retrieved 12/5/18

[450] Black Pepper: www.anniesremedy.com/piper-nigrum-black-pepper.php Retrieved 12/20/18

[451] Blessed Thistle: www.anniesremedy.com/cnicus-benedictus-blessed-thistle.php Retrieved 12/20/18

[452] Blumea: www.stuartxchange.org/Damong-mabaho.html Retrieved 12/5/18

[453] Blumea Camphor: www.stuartxchange.org/Sambong.html Retrieved 12/5/18

[454] Elephant's Foot (E. scaber): www.stuartxchange.org/DilaDila.html Retrieved 12/5/18

[455] Buckwheat: http://whfoods.com/genpage.php?tname=foodspice &dbid=11 Retrieved 3/8/19

[456] Cucumber: http://whfoods.com/genpage.php?tname=foodspice &dbid=42 Retrieved 3/8/19

[457] Goji Berry: www.draxe.com/goji/berry/benefits/ Retrieved 3/8/19

[458] Honey: https://draxe.com/the-many-health-benefits-of-raw-honey/ Retrieved 4/1/19

[459] Lima beans: www.stuartxchange.org/Patani.html Retrieved 12/5/18

[460] Beta-Sitosterol: https://en.wikipedia.org/wiki/Beta-Sitosterol Retrieved 6/30/19 https://www.livestrong.com/article/219561-natural-sources-of-beta-sitosterol/ Retrieved 6/30/19

[461] Piperine: https://www.ncbi.nlm.nih.gov/pubmed/24819444 Retrieved 6/30/19

[462] Flavonoids in Foods: Bhagwat, S., Haytowitz, D.B. Holden, J.M. (Ret.). 2014. USDA Database for the Flavonoid Content of Selected Foods, Release 3.1. U.S. Department of Agriculture, Agricultural Research Service. Nutrient Data Laboratory Home Page: http://www.ars.usda.gov/nutrientdata/flav

[463] Arctigenin: https://en.wikipedia.org/wiki/Arctigenin Retrieved 6/30/19

[464] Betalain: https://en.wikipedia.org/wiki/Betalain Retrieved 6/30/19

[465] Betulinic acid: https://en.wikipedia.org/wiki/ Betulinic_acid Retrieved 6/30/19

[466] Carvone: https://en.wikipedia.org/wiki/Carvone Retrieved 6/30/19

[467] Caryophellene: https://en.wikipedia.org/wiki/ Caryophellene Retrieved 6/30/19

[468] Chicoric acid: https://en.wikipedia.org/wiki/ Chicoric_acid Retrieved 6/30/19

[469] Chlorogenic acid: https://en.wikipedia.org/wiki/ Chlorogenic_acid Retrieved 6/30/19

[470] Cineol: https://en.wikipedia.org/wiki/Eucalyptol Retrieved 6/30/19

[471] Cucurbitacins: http://whfoods.com/genpage.php?tname=foodspice &dbid=42 Retrieved 3/8/19

[472] Ellagic acid: https://en.wikipedia.org/wiki/ Ellagic_acid Retrieved

6/30/19

[473] Ferulic acid: https://en.wikipedia.org/wiki/ Ferulic_acid Retrieved 6/30/19 * http://whfoods.com/genpage.php?tname=foodspice &dbid=45 Retrieved 3/8/19

[474] Genistein: https://en.wikipedia.org/wiki/ Genistein Retrieved 6/30/19

[475] Glucosinolates: https://en.wikipedia.org/wiki/ Glucosinolates Retrieved 6/30/19

[476] Indole-3-carbinol: https://en.wikipedia.org/wiki/ Indole_3_carbinol Retrieved 6/30/19

[477] Inulin: https://en.wikipedia.org/wiki/Inulin Retrieved 6/30/19

[478] Lupeol: https://en.wikipedia.org/wiki/Lupeol Retrieved 6/30/19

[479] Gallic acid: https://en.wikipedia.org/wiki/ Gallic_acid Retrieved 6/30/19

[480] Oleic acid: https://en.wikipedia.org/wiki/ Oleic_acid Retrieved 6/30/19

[481] Palmitic acid: https://en.wikipedia.org/wiki/ Palmitic_acid Retrieved 6/30/19

[482] Pectin: https://en.wikipedia.org/wiki/Pectin Retrieved 6/30/19

[483] Perillyl alcohol: https://en.wikipedia.org/wiki/ Perillyl_alcohol Retrieved 6/30/19

[484] Phytoestrogen: https://en.wikipedia.org/wiki/Phytoestrogen Retrieved 6/30/19

[485] Piceatannol: https://en.wikipedia.org/wiki/Piceatannol Retrieved 6/30/19

[486] Squalene: https://en.wikipedia.org/wiki/Squalene Retrieved 6/30/19

[487] Sulforaphane: https://en.wikipedia.org/wiki/Sulforaphane Retrieved 6/30/19

[488] Ursolic acid: https://en.wikipedia.org/wiki/Ursolic_acid Retrieved 6/30/19

[489] Buckwheat: http://whfoods.com/genpage.php?tname=foodspice &dbid=11 Retrieved 3/8/19

[490] Lovett-Brown, Anna, https://www.herballegacy.com/Lovett-Brown_ Chemical.html Retrieved 12/20/18 * https://articles.mercola.com/ quercetin/ Retrieved 10/16/18

[491] Apricot: http://whfoods.com/genpage.php?tname=foodspice&dbid=3 Retrieved 3/8/19

[492] Arugula: https://draxe.com/arugula/ Retrieved 9/10/18

[493] Betaine and Betalains: https://draxe.com/what-is-betaine/ Retrieved on 08-20-2018 * https://en.wikipedia.org/wiki/Indicaxanthin Retrieved on 08-16-2018

[494] Blueberry: ttp://whfoods.com/genpage.php?tname=foodspice&dbid=8 Retrieved 3/8/19 * https://draxe.com/pterostilbene/ Retrieved 3/8/19

[495] Butternut Squash: www.draxe.com/butternut-squash-nutrition/ Retrieved 3/16/19

[496] Oligosaccharides: https://en.wikipedia.org/wiki/Fructans Retrieved on 08-16-2018

[497] Oat Beta-Glucs: http://en.wikipedia.org/Oat_beta-glucan